W9-DFI-764

NEAL'S YARD REMEDIES

Make your Own
Cosmetics

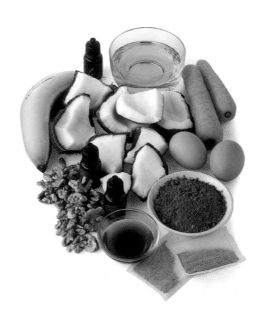

Make your Own
Cosmetics

Recipes • Skin Care • Body Care • Hair Care
Perfumes & Fragrancing • Herbs • Essential Oils
Cosmetic Ingredients • Useful Addresses

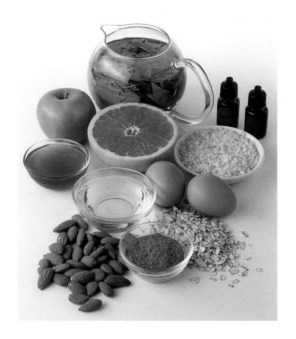

AURUM PRESS

First published in the UK in 1997 by
Aurum Press Ltd
25 Bedford Avenue
London WC1B 3AT

ISBN: 1-85410-469-1

Colour reproduction by Monarch, Bristol, England

Printed in Singapore

A HALDANE MASON BOOK

Conceived, designed and produced by Haldane Mason, London

Editorial: Diana Vowles,
Lydia Darbyshire, Christopher Fagg
Photography: Amanda Heywood
Illustrator: Stephen Dew

For Neal's Yard Remedies: Gill Armstrong, Susan Curtis, Romy Fraser, Pauline Hili,
Lara Loxley, Vivienne Palmer, Vikki Prevett, Alice Rhodes

Thanks also to Sydney Francis, all NYR staff who helped test the products and the
NYR Design department for their help and support.

Neal's Yard Remedies and the publishers have made every effort to test the recipes
contained in this book. However, they cannot be held responsible for adverse
reactions to any products made by members of the public. A patch test should be
carried out before any cosmetic preparation is used.

Contents

Foreword

At the beginning of 1981 I decided to set up an apothecary shop in Neal's Yard, Covent Garden. It took almost a year to design the shop, source the products and get everything ready for the opening in December. One of the key aims was to create hair and skin products that really worked and that did what they said they would do, but in such a way that didn't involve a long chain of processes during which the beneficial effects of natural ingredients were lost.

Recipes for the care of the body can be found dating back many centuries, and I'm sure that even before recipes were recorded by the ancient Egyptians, Greeks and Romans, people would have been well acquainted with ways of looking after themselves by using the resources they found in their local environment.

Health and beauty products tend to be localized. Pumice can be obtained from volcanic areas; herbs containing saponins are used for cleansing in the Amazon; colourings are derived from roots and animals in various parts of the world. Traditional recipes have been developed from these ingredients. Men and women have always been concerned with the way they look, using ingredients to shine their hair, polish their nails, perfume their bodies and delay the onset of the ageing process.

It is only relatively recently that people have lost the ability and the desire to make their own hair and skin products from plants, animals and minerals. Increasingly complex processes have been developed during this century to produce commercial products, and most people do not know what ingredients are used. Detergents, preservatives, stabilizers, colourings, artificial fragrances and petroleum by-products are more common than not. They may not be harmful to your skin or hair, but they are probably not very friendly to the environment.

While developing the products for the first Neal's Yard Remedies, I realized that there had to be a compromise. The customers I anticipated using the products wouldn't always be inclined to wash their hair in two stages, using a soap-based shampoo, which is alkaline, followed by an acid conditioning rinse. People expect creams to last indefinitely and are not prepared to go to the refrigerator to look for a face cream. The products, therefore, needed to contain preservatives and emulsifiers to keep creams and lotions from separating, and detergents seemed inevitable. Returning to the past didn't seem to be an option, as we clearly needed to sell products that people would use. However, the policy of Neal's Yard Remedies has always been to make products that do not contain colourings, artificial fragrances or petrochemical ingredients.

A few years after the shop was set up we became uneasy that real purists weren't catered for, so a corner was set aside to stock ingredients that, with the right information, would enable anyone to make their own skin and hair care products. That section is still there, complemented from time to time by

recipes that cus-
tomers can take
away and try. It
soon became obvious, however,
that we needed a good book for people
to use as a reference and source of ideas.

I confess that I don't often make my own skin creams, but in the course of preparing this book, many of us in the company found ourselves involved in the process of creating mixtures and lotions to include. All those ideas that we've had for products but have never found space on the shelves are in this book! We've also included recipes for some of the products that are sold in our shops.

There are huge benefits to be gained from making your own creams. First, you can adjust them to to suit your own skin type. As your skill in making creams and lotions develops and your knowledge of herbs and oils widens, so will your ability to make products specific to your needs, whether they be creams, deodorants or foot powders. Second, you can control the ingredients you use. At the moment we have very little idea of what goes into products, and even the more informative labelling to be enforced by EU legislation in January 1998 will not mean much to anyone but a cosmetic scientist. Third, there are fashions and trends in fragrances, yet everybody is unique. It can be an enjoyable process to discover the fragrances that suit your mood and the image you want to project, and making your own products allows you to do this.

A further benefit is that the process of making the products is creative. Being creative can often involve different skills from those you normally use on a daily basis. Performing repetitive tasks makes people uncreative and unstimulated, and such a life is also stressful. Being involved in any creative process can help you unwind and give a sense of achievement and of being yourself after a frustrating day.

You can involve children in making home products. It is comparatively easy, it is fun, and they will learn about the healing properties of herbs and oils and gain skills in measuring and recording. Use this book to enjoy making your own recipes. Don't be restricted to the recipes that are listed – use them as ideas.

Lastly, and perhaps more subtly, working with natural ingredients puts you in touch with the natural environment. It is best to use fresh herbs. Many, like sage and rosemary, are often grown for cooking. Learn to grow comfrey and marigolds and plant some lavender or lemon balm in a flower tub or window box.

This book has been a group effort. Our product development team has tried out hundreds of ideas. Everyone in the company has become used to the aromas of boiling herbs in the reception area, trays of soap drying out in the kitchen and bottles of lotions and packs of powders appearing on our desks to try out. The process has drawn in everyone at Neal's Yard Remedies, and I hope this involvement will be extended to the readers of this book.

Romy Fraser, Managing Director,
Neal's Yard Remedies, London, March 1997

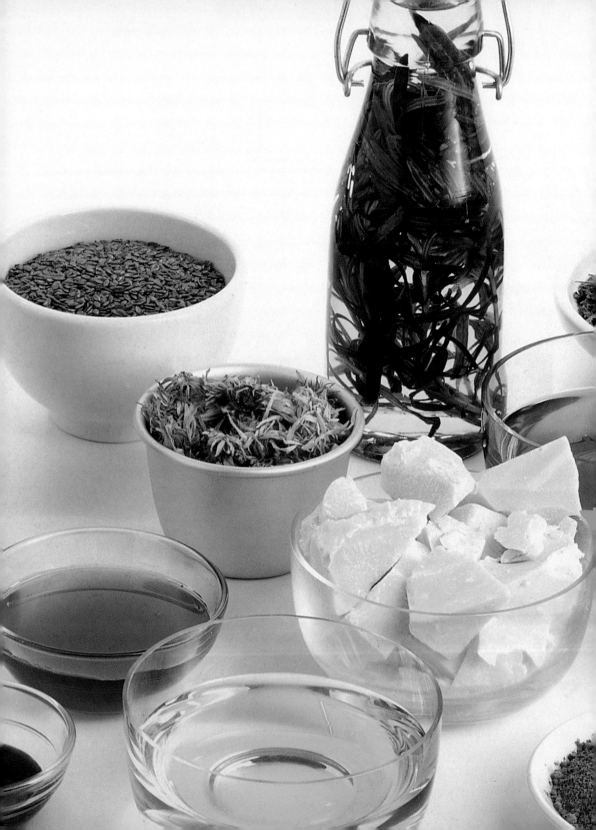

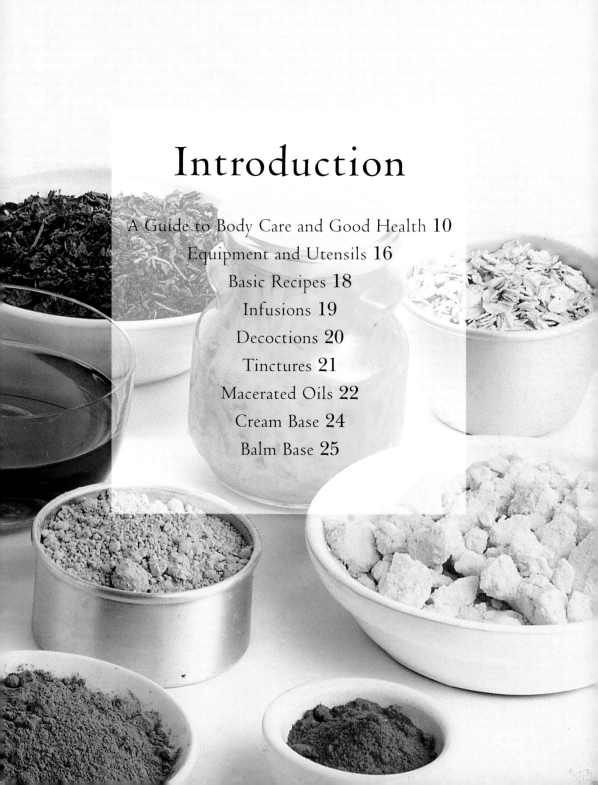

Introduction

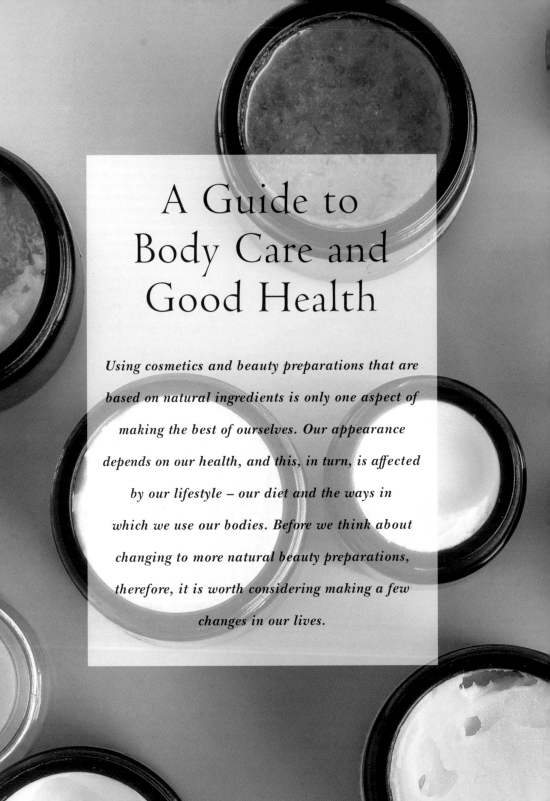

A Guide to Body Care and Good Health

Using cosmetics and beauty preparations that are based on natural ingredients is only one aspect of making the best of ourselves. Our appearance depends on our health, and this, in turn, is affected by our lifestyle – our diet and the ways in which we use our bodies. Before we think about changing to more natural beauty preparations, therefore, it is worth considering making a few changes in our lives.

This book is about beauty, and beauty depends so much upon our energy, how we feel about ourselves, and how comfortable we are with our body. Not all of us have the super-slim, boyish look that is currently promoted by the fashion and media industries, but we can all take positive steps to improve our level of health and self-esteem. A healthy, smiling, radiant face will always have an inherent beauty, whether or not the individual features making up that face conform to our preconceived ideas of attractiveness.

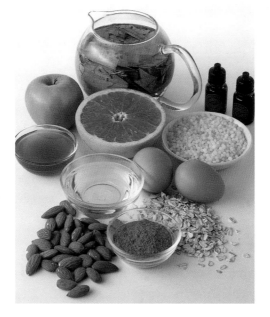

To enjoy good health and to feel energetic we need to look after the spiritual, mental and emotional aspects of our lives as well as our physical health. There is a flow of energy between these different aspects of ourselves, and this integrates and keeps us healthy and whole.

All the processes of life and nature are interconnected: in order for a meadow to produce sweet healthy grass, for example, the soil must be fertile, the river and rainwater must be pure, and the meadow must be managed with an understanding of the natural cycles involved in creating good pasture. You cannot separate one part from the whole and expect it to remain healthy in isolation, and similarly you cannot expect to have healthy, clear skin without taking your general level of health into account.

The underlying causes of skin disease can be difficult to unravel, and they are generally a complex combination of diet, environment, general health, hereditary factors, stress and individual susceptibility. Coping with a skin problem without suppressing it with strong medication is a real challenge for many people who would like to make the decision to switch to a more natural approach to life and health.

A psychological approach to dealing with skin problems might include meditation, visualization, counselling or any of the other methods that are available to help with stress.

The link between the mind and emotions and the skin is a very complex one. If we have a skin problem it can be very difficult not to feel self-conscious about it, and not to let it dent our self-confidence. On the other hand, many of us find that our skin condition is affected by the amount of stress we are experiencing, creating a vicious cycle. For some contacts on psychological approaches and other complementary therapies see the Useful Addresses on page 138.

ENVIRONMENT

The main functions of the skin include protection and elimination. The more toxic the external and internal environment, the harder the skin has to work. If the load becomes too great the skin will begin to show signs of disease. Unfortunately, we live in an increasingly toxic world, and as a result a wide range of allergies, sensitivities and diseases of many kinds are on the increase.

It is easy to feel overwhelmed by the number of toxins to which we are exposed, but there are several steps that may be taken to minimize the impact that they may have. Identifying the more immediate hazards and choosing to do something about them can be a very empowering process. Some that we do have the ability to change are smoking, drinking alcohol, eating adulterated foods, taking drugs, wearing synthetic fibres and using chemical-laden toiletries and cosmetics. Other factors, such as environmental pollution and radiation, may seem beyond our control, but even here there are measures that each of us can take in order to cut down on exposure and minimize risks.

HOW TO IMPROVE YOUR ENVIRONMENT

- Make sure any rooms you live or work in for lengthy periods of time are well ventilated.

- If you have air-conditioning units make sure that they are serviced regularly.

- If your living rooms have double-glazing and central heating the air can be very drying, so install a humidifier or buy plenty of plants.

- A build-up of positive ions can lead to feelings of lethargy and lowered vitality. Install an ionizer in any room containing a lot of electrical equipment such as televisions and computers.

- Make the most of natural daylight. Our nervous systems need full-spectrum light to maintain health, so if you are in artificial light for prolonged periods install full-spectrum lighting.

- Filter heavy metals and nitrates out of tap water for drinking and cooking.

- Green houseplants help to decrease carbon dioxide and benzene fumes.

- Choose natural furnishings such as wood, cotton and wool rather than synthetics.

- Use non-toxic paint when decorating and natural paper wall coverings rather than synthetic ones.

- Use natural flooring materials, such as ceramic tiles, cork or wood and natural fibres, such as wool, coir or cotton, rather than synthetic fibre carpets.

- Avoid using aerosols – as well as damaging the atmosphere they give off a fine mist of chemicals that are easily absorbed by the lungs and skin.

- Ask your dentist for porcelain or plastic fillings rather than amalgam ones, which contain toxic mercury.

- Use anti-glare screens on computers to reduce the positive ion effect.

FOOD

The phrase 'you are what you eat' has been understood by healers since ancient times, but in recent decades we seem to have lost sight of it. Hippocrates (460–377 BC) outlined some illuminating truths about food, including: 'Let food be your medicine and let medicine be your food.' This illustrates very clearly how important our diet and eating habits are to our overall health.

If we eat refined, processed and polluted foods, we cannot expect to be healthy. In addition, since one of the primary functions of the skin is as an organ of elimination, if we eat foods that are laden with chemicals that our body has to clear out we must expect to have unhealthy-looking skin.

So what kind of food should we eat? Basically, the closer it is to its original state the more food retains its nutritional value. Food needs to be as fresh and as unprocessed and unrefined as possible. Ideally, we should eat as much of the whole product as possible, as with brown rice or wholemeal flour.

Refined foods are often low in vitamins, and to compensate for this, some foods actually have vitamins added. This seems rather a waste of resources. However, the fact that intensive agricultural methods have caused a decline in the natural vitamins and minerals in our food may mean that some of us will need to take food supplements. There is no substitute for good, fresh food, but if you feel that some supplement is necessary, choose an additive-free, well-balanced supplement or consult a nutritional advisor.

In the post-war period, factory farming was developed to increase the self-sufficiency of the nation and to provide cheaper food. However, there have been some alarming incidents in recent years to indicate that we need to reassess our attitude to producing food. The battery farming of chickens has led to outbreaks of salmonella bacteria in eggs and poultry. Feeding cows on an unnatural diet of meat products is implicated in the development of BSE, a disease for which our poor understanding of nature is responsible. The overuse of nitrates in agricultural practices has led to the pollution of our water.

We are now having to accept irradiated food as an alternative to fresh food. Several supermarkets offer irradiated soft fruit for sale because of its increased keeping properties, and they do not have to indicate its status. In 1996 the first genetically modified soya beans arrived in Europe from the USA, and 60 per cent of the food we eat contains soya or its derivatives. This is despite the fact that the potential health implications such as increased food allergies have not been researched.

Nevertheless, there are some steps we can take towards improving the quality of the food we eat and these are summarized overleaf.

If you are aware that you have not had a very good diet for some years, or that your diet is contributing to a particular disease, you could consider consulting a dietary therapist or a naturopath for specific advice. The naturopathic approach to health is that we need to be able to clear out impurities or toxins in our system, rather than letting them build up and contribute to disease. If we are reasonably healthy we should be able to eliminate a small amount of additives and toxins naturally, through our bowels, bladder and skin. However, if the level of toxins in our diet is too high, or if our eliminative processes are blocked or under-functioning, symptoms of disease will result.

IMPROVING THE QUALITY OF OUR DIET

* Where possible, store food in glass or china containers, not in plastic or clingfilm (plastic wrap), which may leach toxic chemicals into your food.

* Avoid using aluminium foil wrappings on acidic food such as fruit or fruit cakes.

* Avoid using aluminium cooking utensils; choose instead glass, stainless steel or high-quality enamel (not chipped).

* Steam or stir-fry vegetables to retain the maximum amount of nutrients.

* Do not use microwaves for any food containing dairy products as the molecular structure of the proteins is altered and the effects of this are unknown. Also avoid heating food covered in plastic wraps which may allow the migration of toxic chemicals into your food.

* Avoid consuming large amounts of salt, refined sugar and animal fats.

* Avoid all food additives – i.e., foods containing E numbers – especially artificial colourings.

* Increase your intake of fresh vegetables, raw food and fruit.

* Where possible buy organically produced food.

A detoxifying or cleansing diet can be a good way to clear out the system, and a good start to making improvements in your diet. The 10-day cleansing diet shown on the opposite page is effective and fairly gentle.

Alternatively, consult a naturopath or dietary therapist who will guide you through a cleansing regime to suit your particular needs. It is traditionally considered to be particularly beneficial to follow a cleansing diet in the spring and/or autumn.

If you have any particular health problem you should consult your health practitioner before going on a special diet.

EXERCISE

Being beautiful and staying healthy goes hand in hand not only with what we eat, but also with keeping fit. This becomes even more true the older we get. Keeping fit does not necessarily mean working out every day or jogging 8 kilometres (5 miles) before breakfast, but it does require a commitment to regular, moderate exercise. The type of exercise that is most likely to be sustained is that which you can build into your daily life and routine, such as walking the kids to school, doing 20 minutes of yoga before lunch and cycling to work. Getting some exercise every day will help you to feel more energetic.

Remember you don't have to develop macho muscles or be super thin to feel good about your body, but regular exercise will help you to feel trimmer, better about your body and better about yourself.

A DETOXIFYING DIET

Day 1	Fruit for breakfast, lunch and in the evening. Choose one type of fruit for each meal from the following: apples, pears or grapes. Eat as much fruit as you like at one sitting.
Day 2	Fruit for breakfast. Choose one type of fruit each day from: apples, pears, grapes, kiwi fruit, tomatoes and grapefruit. Eat raw vegetables for lunch. Make a mixture of at least five salad vegetables: mix roots (carrots, grated beetroot and so on), sprouts and leafy vegetables. In the evening, eat cooked vegetables. Make a soup by boiling a mixture of at least five vegetables, preferably including onions. Do not add any salt or seasoning.
Day 3	See Day 2.
Day 4	See Day 2.
Day 5	See Day 2.
Day 6	See Day 2.
Day 7	Breakfast: as Day 2. Lunch: as Day 2, but in addition eat two pieces of dry crispbread or two rice cakes. Evening: as Day 2.
Day 8	See Day 7.
Day 9	See Day 7.
Day 10	Breakfast: as Day 2. Lunch: as Day 7. Evening: as Day 2, but in addition eat a baked potato with a small knob of butter.

* Drink plenty of mineral water every day, and eat as much organically produced fruit and vegetables as possible.

* It is not unusual to get symptoms such as headaches, tiredness and skin eruptions during a cleansing diet. This is an indication that toxins are being released from the tissues and into the bloodstream before they are eliminated. If you drink enough water these symptoms usually disappear in a day or two.

* Important things to avoid altogether throughout the diet are tea, coffee, cigarettes, salt, sugar, pepper, drugs, alcohol, antiperspirants and late nights.

Equipment and Utensils

Very little specialized equipment is required to make the recipes in this book, and most of the utensils needed will be found in the average kitchen. Before you begin to make any of the products, read quickly through the recipe to check that you have everything you will need. The list below summarizes the items used, but you can, of course, improvise with your own kitchen utensils.

If you do not have a bain-marie, place the ingredients to be heated in a heatproof bowl that will sit on the rim of a saucepan that is one-quarter to one-third filled with water. As the water is heated, the bowl becomes warm and the warmth will permeate to the ingredients and soften them.

Jars that are sold for homemade preserves are ideal for storing many of the recipes, and good cookware stores supply a range of sizes. Look out especially for the smaller ones. These jars have sealable lids that are held in place by metal clips, which create an airtight seal. Some types also have rubber rings around the lids, which provide an even tighter seal. Creams and balms are best stored in dark-coloured glass jars and bottles.

Before you begin, sterilize all the equipment you need, including the boxes and bottles (and their lids) that will hold the finished product, by immersing them in boiling water for 20 minutes. Remember, too, to wash your hands thoroughly before you start.

BASIC KIT

- Atomizer spray
- Bain-marie or double saucepan
- Bun tin (cookie pan)
- Clingfilm (plastic kitchen film)
- Coffee filter (unbleached)
- Fork
- Funnel
- Glass bowls (at least two sizes)

- Glass jars and bottles (various sizes)
- Grater
- Hand whisk
- Kettle
- Knife
- Labels and pen
- Measuring jug
- Muslin (cheesecloth)

- Pestle and mortar
- Saucepan
- Screw-top or sealable jars
- Spoons (wooden and metal)
- Strainer or sieve
- Tea pot
- Teaspoon and tablespoon or measuring spoons

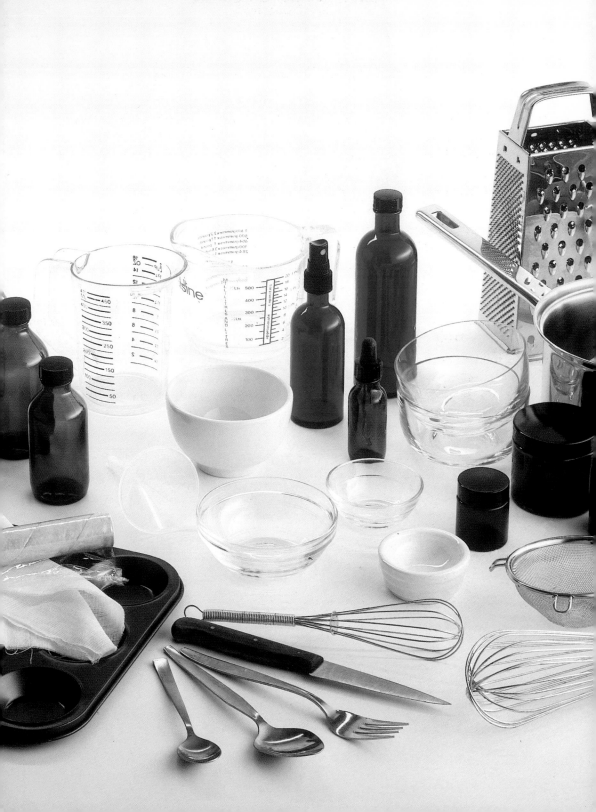

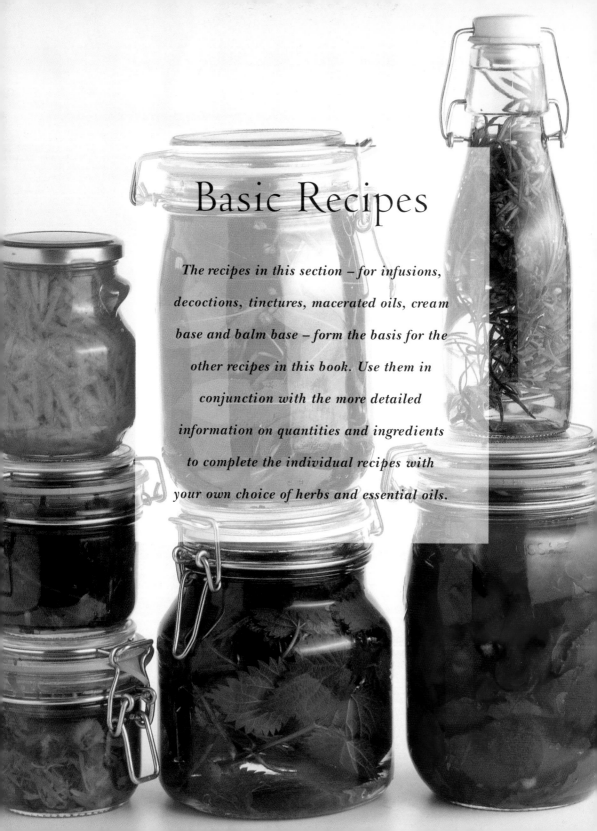

Basic Recipes

The recipes in this section – for infusions, decoctions, tinctures, macerated oils, cream base and balm base – form the basis for the other recipes in this book. Use them in conjunction with the more detailed information on quantities and ingredients to complete the individual recipes with your own choice of herbs and essential oils.

Infusions

An infusion is made like a tea. It is the appropriate way to harness the properties of the softer, green or flowering parts of a plant. Infusions are very easy to make. They can be used instead of water in any of the recipes in this book and are a simple way of including a specific herb for a particular skin type or condition.

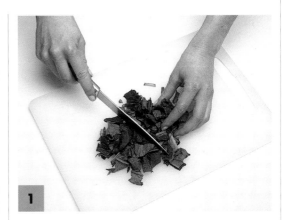

QUANTITY

The quantity of herb varies according to the herb used, the strength of infusion required and its desired purpose. Unless otherwise stated, the standard measurement is 1 heaped teaspoon of dried herb to 1 cup of boiling water. Wherever possible use fresh herbs and double the quantity. For a simple infusion with increased effectiveness, add more herb.

1 Chop the herb or mixture of herbs. Transfer to a cup or teapot.

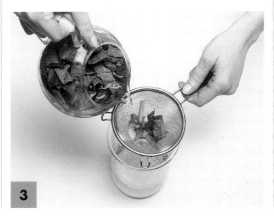

2 Pour on boiling water. Leave to steep for 10 minutes, preferably covered to avoid the loss of volatile oils in the steam.

3 Strain before use. Make up as required.

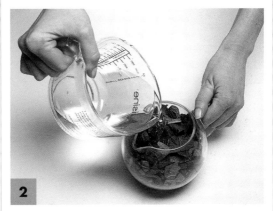

Herbs that can be easily used in infusions include:

Borage • Chamomile • Cleavers • Comfrey leaf
Elderflower • Lavender • Lemon balm
Marigold • Marsh mallow leaf • Rose petals

Decoctions

This is the appropriate way to use the woodier parts of a plant – its roots, bark, berries and seeds. Decoctions should be prepared on the day they are used.

1 Place the herb or mixture of herbs in a saucepan. Try to avoid using an aluminium one.

2 Pour on water, cover and bring to the boil. Simmer for 10 minutes. Strain before use.

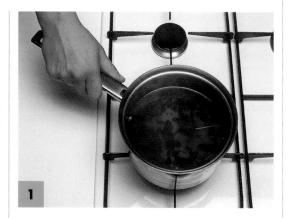

QUANTITY

The quantity of herb varies according to the herb used, the strength of decoction required and its desired purpose. Unless otherwise stated, the standard measurement is 1 heaped teaspoon of dried herb to 1 cup of boiling water. You may need to add more water if steam escapes. Where possible use fresh herbs and double the quantity.

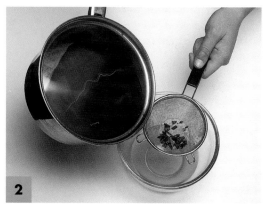

Herbs that can be used in decoctions include:

Burdock root • Echinacea • Fennel • Ginseng
Marsh mallow root • Quassia

Always label the products you make with the name and date of making.

Tinctures

The medicinal properties of a herb can be extracted using alcohol. The alcohol also acts as a preservative, making this an excellent way to store herbs out of season. It is standard practice to use one herb per tincture, although it is possible to combine tinctures. Tinctures will keep for up to 12 months.

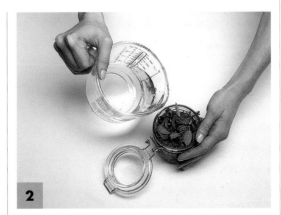

1 Pack a sealable jar tightly with finely chopped herbs, preferably fresh.

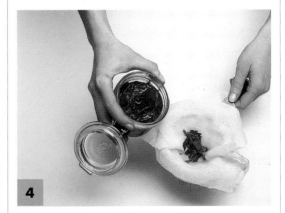

2 Immerse the herb totally in vodka and water. Refer to the list of ratios, which vary for each herb (see pages 136–137). Note that the final volume is based on 100% proof alcohol (available from duty-free shops); we therefore recommend using high-proof vodka.

3 Seal the jar and store for 2 weeks away from direct sunlight, shaking occasionally.

4 Strain the mixture through muslin (cheesecloth) and then filter through an unbleached coffee filter.

5 Pour into a dark glass bottle. Label clearly with the name and date, and store in a cool place away from sunlight.

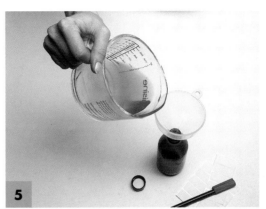

Herbs that can be used in tinctures include:

Borage • Cleavers • Lemon balm • Marigold
Nettle • Sage • Yarrow

Macerated Oils

The volatile oils contained in aromatic plants can be released by soaking them in vegetable oil. This is called an infused or macerated oil. Macerated oils can be used as carrier oils or they can be incorporated into cosmetic recipes. There are two methods of preparation.

METHOD 1
THE SUN METHOD

This method can also be used with cider vinegar or witch hazel instead of vegetable oil. The oil will keep for up to 12 months.

1 Pack a sealable jar tightly with finely chopped fresh herbs.

2 Cover the herbs with a good-quality vegetable oil. Virgin olive oil and sweet almond oil are best, although sunflower oil is a good alternative. It is very important that the plant material is completely covered by the oil both for full extraction and to exclude contamination.

3 Seal the jar and leave in direct sunlight for 2 weeks, shaking daily.

4 Strain and repeat with fresh plant material. Leave for another 2 weeks, shaking daily.

5 Strain, pour into a dark glass bottle and label with the name and date.

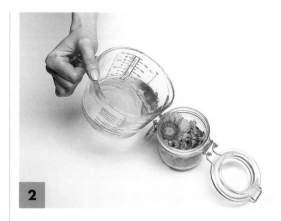

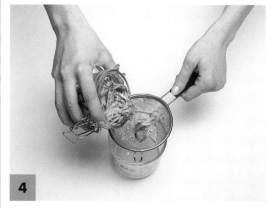

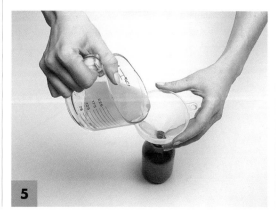

Macerated Oils

THE HEATING METHOD

This method is faster and possibly more practical, especially if the oil is needed for immediate use. The oil will keep for up to 12 months.

1 Place the finely chopped herbs in a bowl.

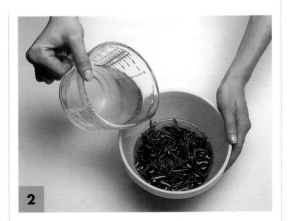

2 Cover with vegetable oil. It is not necessary to use cold-pressed oil as heating the oil ruins the benefits of that type of extraction.

3 Place the bowl containing the mixture over a pan of boiling water and heat for 1 hour.

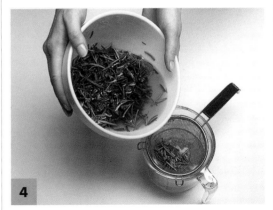

4 Remove from the heat, strain and repeat with fresh herbs.

5 Strain, pour into a dark glass bottle and label with the name and date.

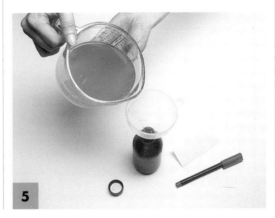

Herbs that can be used in macerates include:

Calendula • Carrot • Comfrey • Garlic
Mullein • St John's Wort

23

Cream Base

This is a simple cream base that can be used to carry essential oils and herbal tinctures for external application. It will keep well in the refrigerator for up to 2 months. The ingredients given here are sufficient to make about 100 g/3½ oz.

8 g/2 tsp beeswax (granules or grated)
10 g cocoa butter
30 ml/2 tbsp almond oil
15 ml/1 tbsp wheatgerm oil
45 ml/1½ fl oz/3 tbsp spring water
½ tsp borax

1 Heat the beeswax, cocoa butter and base oils together in a bowl over a saucepan of water until the ingredients have melted.

2 Warm the spring water in a saucepan and dissolve the borax in it.

3 Take the oily mixture off the heat. Slowly add the spring water mixture to the oily mixture and stir until cool.

4 Add the essential oils or herbal tincture. Store in a dark glass jar in the refrigerator.

VARIATIONS
You can replace the spring water with an infusion, which will allow you to include herbs that suit your own skin type and skin requirements. You could also substitute other oils of your choice for the almond or wheatgerm oils.

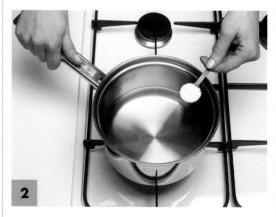

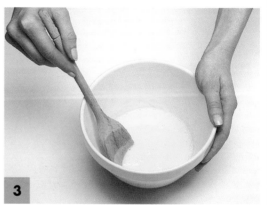

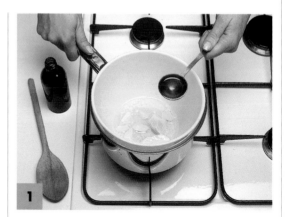

Balm Base

This is a simple base that does not use borax. It works well, but does not have the creamy texture of the previous recipe. It can set quite hard, depending on the ratio of beeswax to oils, and will last for 6 months if it is stored in an airtight jar. The ingredients given here are sufficient to make about 100 g/3½ oz.

8 g/2 tsp beeswax (granules or grated)
45 ml/3 tbsp almond oil
15 ml/1 tbsp wheatgerm oil
10 ml/2 tsp herb tincture
5 drops essential oil

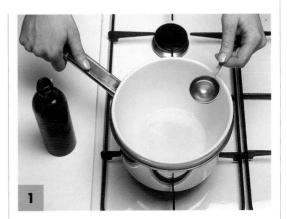

1 Heat the beeswax and almond oil in a bowl over a saucepan of boiling water until the beeswax has melted.

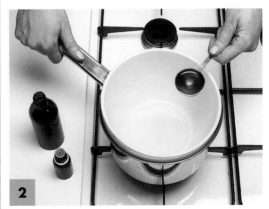

2 Add the wheatgerm oil and tincture and gently stir together. Remove from the heat and allow to cool slightly.

3 Add the essential oils and mix thoroughly. Pour into a dark glass jar and allow to set.

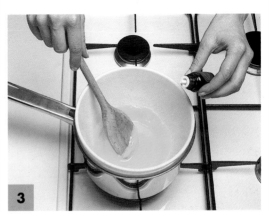

VARIATIONS

As with the Cream Base, you can use oils of your choice instead of the almond and wheatgerm oils. It is an ideal recipe to use for making up first-aid remedies. If you learn the properties of the herbs you will discover that there is an endless range of opportunities available.

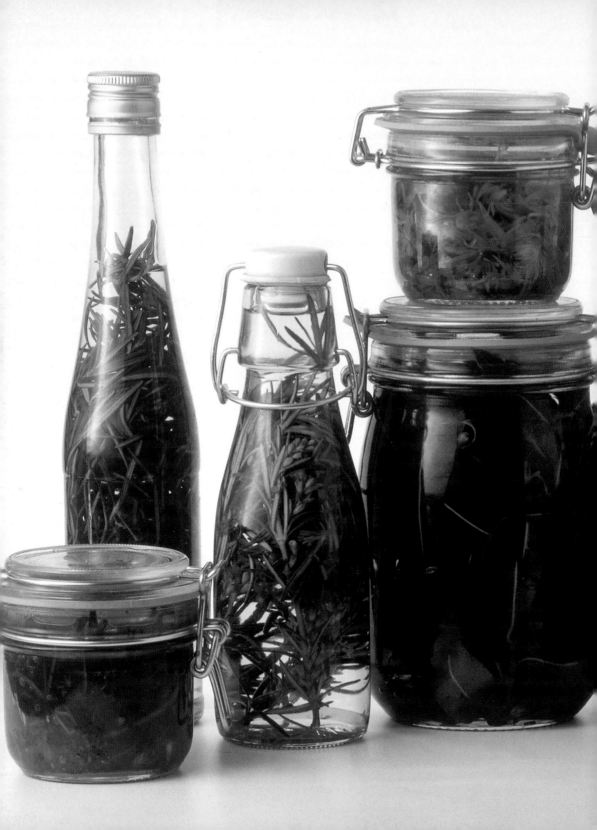

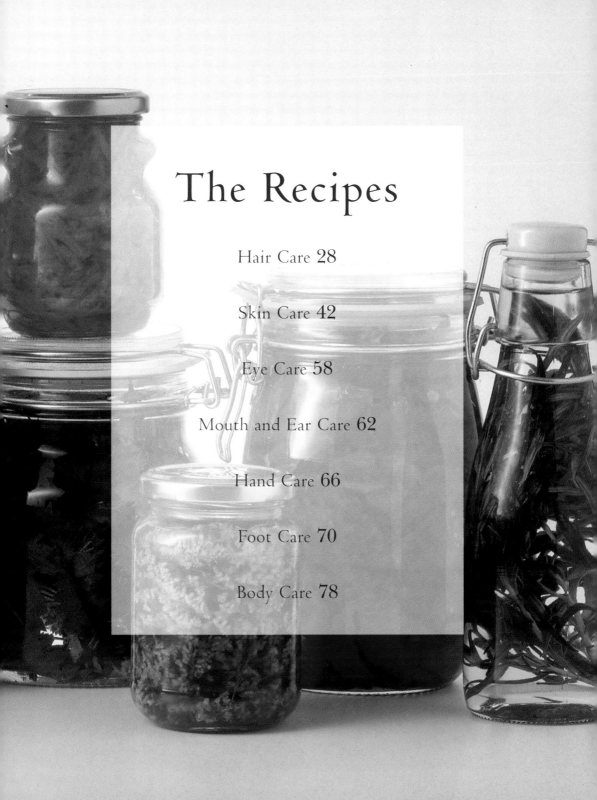

The Recipes

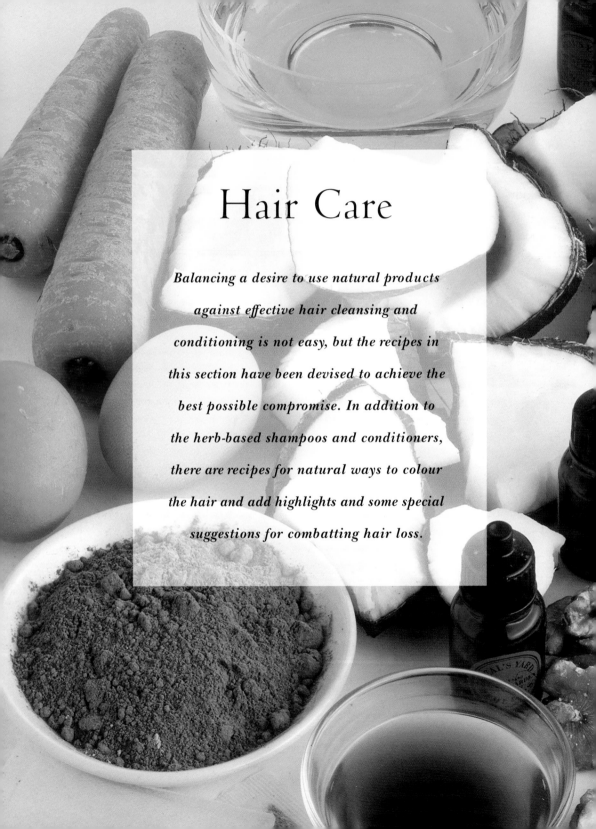

Hair Care

Balancing a desire to use natural products against effective hair cleansing and conditioning is not easy, but the recipes in this section have been devised to achieve the best possible compromise. In addition to the herb-based shampoos and conditioners, there are recipes for natural ways to colour the hair and add highlights and some special suggestions for combatting hair loss.

There are dozens of hair-care products on the market today, and selecting an appropriate one is often a difficult process that can be avoided by making your own at home. A typical routine for developing and maintaining beautiful hair consists of shampooing, conditioning, scalp massage and the use of treatments and finishing products. Few of us, however, have the time to perform all of these tasks on a regular basis, and we generally limit hair care to washing and conditioning.

When you are making your own hair-care products, it is useful to know how each type of preparation works. The primary aim of shampooing is, of course, to remove dirt from the hair. This dirt consists mainly of bodily secretions, but atmospheric dust and pollutants and residues from hair-grooming preparations also need to be cleaned away. An effective shampoo removes grease and water-soluble dirt without stripping away all the natural oiliness of the hair. The active cleansing ingredient in shampoos is known as a surfactant, which functions by removing the dirt from the hair surface and dispersing it in the washing solution so that it is not redeposited on the clean hair or scalp. Surfactants are commonly known as detergents.

The earliest shampoos contained soap, but today they are generally based on non-soap detergents. Detergents are a synthetically produced group of chemicals, and although they are often based on a natural material, such as coconut oil or palm kernel oil, they are generally highly modified. This causes one of the most difficult formulation dilemmas for those of us committed to producing a highly natural product. A shampoo based on soap would create dull and damaged-looking hair when used over a long period unless much time and effort were taken to condition the hair. Modern shampoos offer a convenience and effectiveness that is difficult to match with totally natural products.

In formulating the Neal's Yard Remedies range of shampoos we have tried to come up with the best compromise. Detergents are used but are balanced by herbs and natural oils, which provide their natural benefits. It is not the ultimate solution, but it is one that allows us to offer our customers convenience while at the same time producing a shampoo containing a large percentage of natural raw materials.

The recipes presented in this section are great for those of us with the time to spend using them correctly. The shampoo bar is a fabulous travelling companion, but make sure that you condition your hair well after use because soaps can be drying on the hair. When you use the dry shampoo base, section your hair before applying it in order to avoid too much clumping of dry materials.

Because of the large proportion of water they contain, homemade shampoos need to be made and stored with care to avoid microbial contamination. It is probably best to make up the shampoo on the day of use.

If you do not have much time to spare but would like to make your own products, you can start with some ordinary shampoo and add your own herbal infusions and essential oils. Because you are diluting the detergent, you will find you have a shampoo that foams less but is much milder on your hair. As a rough guide the following ratio is recommended:

50 per cent ordinary shampoo –
   e.g. 50 ml/3¼ tbsp
45 per cent herbal infusion –
   e.g. 45 ml/1½ fl oz/3 tbsp
4 per cent natural oils (jojoba, coconut) –
   e.g. 4 ml/1 scant tsp
0.2–1 per cent essential oils –
   e.g. 0.2–1 ml/4–20 drops

Whichever product you decide suits you, remember to pay attention to what your hair is telling you. If it starts to look lank and dull, make some changes to your favourite formula to achieve a better result. Hormonal and environmental factors will influence the feel and look of your hair, and you may have to adapt formulae that once worked well for you.

Hair conditioner is much easier to achieve naturally than shampoo, and the range of materials is also greater. The active ingredients in commercial conditioners are known as cationic surfactants. After shampooing, hair is often left without sufficient natural oil, and conditioners aim to repair this. The cationic surfactants in conventional conditioners are attracted to damaged hair where keratin has been affected and a negative charge has built up. This results in overall improvement to the condition of the hair.

Using a herb rinse is a great way of achieving the same results as conventional conditioners with homemade ones. Use the chart opposite to select the herb that is suitable for your hair type. Make an infusion (see page 19) and add to it some fresh fruit juice, glycerine and lecithin.

Before synthetic detergents were invented, rinses of lemon juice or cider vinegar were used to improve the shine and feel of the hair after washing. Both materials are acidic, help to soften the water and have an astringent effect on the hair, shrinking the cuticles and making the shaft smoother. If your hair tends to be greasy, use a water-based product; if it is dry, choose an oil-based one. The recipes provided here give both options.

There are some excellent, easily available conditioning bases, which can be used on their own or combined with other ingredients, including beer, eggs, milk and natural oils such as jojoba and coconut.

Many of the recipes in this section may be adapted to suit your own hair type. The essential oils and herbal infusions on the opposite page may be substituted for ingredients listed where appropriate.

HAIR TYPE	ESSENTIAL OILS	HERBAL INFUSIONS
NORMAL	Cedarwood, lavender, orange, rosemary	Rose, rosemary, thyme
OILY	Bergamot, cedarwood, cypress, geranium, grapefruit, juniper, lemon, lime, petitgrain	Elderflower, lemon balm, mint, rosemary, sage, yarrow
DRY	Olibanum, palmarosa, sandalwood	Calendula, chamomile, marsh mallow, oat straw
DAMAGED	Comfrey, horsetail, lavender, olibanum, seaweed	Calendula, coltsfoot
DULL	Melissa, rosemary	Ginseng, horsetail, nettle, rosemary, sage
FINE	Geranium	Calendula, oat straw
DARK	Rosemary, thyme	Nettle, rosemary, thyme
FAIR	Roman chamomile	Chamomile, mullein flowers
GREY	Sage	Rosemary, sage
FREQUENT WASH	Geranium, horsetail, lavender, rosemary	Coltsfoot, elderflower, seaweed
CHILDREN	Roman chamomile	Chamomile, rose
DANDRUFF	Cedarwood, patchouli, rosemary, sage, tea tree, thyme	Chamomile, elderflower, nettle, sage

Shampoos

YO-JOJOBA AND A BOTTLE OF RUM

An excellent pre-shampoo treatment and hair tonic. These ingredients make enough for one treatment.

5 ml/1 tsp rum
5 ml/1 tsp jojoba oil
5 ml/1 tsp liquid lecithin
4 drops essential oil of your choice

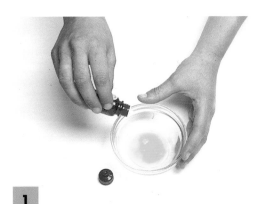

1

1 Blend all the ingredients together, then massage over your head and scalp.

2 Wrap a towel around your head and leave for 1 hour.

3 Wash out, using a mild shampoo with lemon juice added.

DRY SHAMPOO BASE

A dry shampoo to freshen up and cleanse your hair when you are in a hurry. See the chart on page 31 for a guide to the use of herbs. These ingredients make enough for one treatment.

1 tsp orris root
2 tsp arrowroot
2 tsp dried herbs

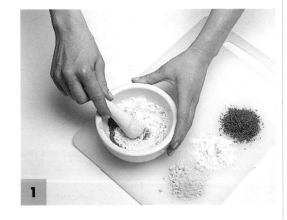

1

1 Mix all the ingredients together and grind to a fine powder in a mortar and pestle.

2 Rub the powder into wet hair and then rinse out.

Shampoos

SAGE SHAMPOO BAR

This handy shampoo bar is useful for travelling. It is most effective on short hair. These ingredients will make about six bars.

1 tsp dried sage
300 ml/½ pt/1¼ cups water
½ bar almond soap
45 ml/3 tbsp vegetable glycerine
10 drops lemon essential oil

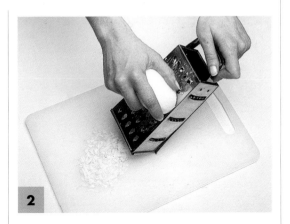

1 Make an infusion (see page 19) using the sage and water and strain it.

2 Grate the soap and add it to the sage infusion. Heat until all the soap has melted.

3 While the mixture is still hot, add the vegetable glycerine. Remove from heat.

4 Add the essential oil, pour the mixture into baking tins and leave uncovered to set.

5 Use the bars as soap. They will keep for 3 weeks in the refrigerator.

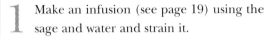

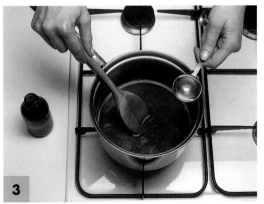

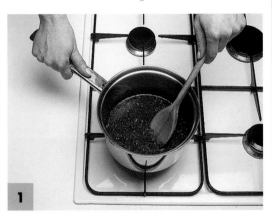

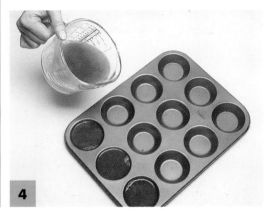

Conditioners

COCONUT CONDITIONER

This recipe is easy to make and is suitable for all hair types, depending on the essential oils used. See the chart on page 31 for a guide to the use of essential oils. These ingredients will make 100 g/3½ oz. It will keep for up to 12 months.

100 g/3½ oz jar coconut oil
20 drops essential oil

1 Melt the coconut oil by standing the jar in a bowl of hot water. Add the essential oils and stir before it re-sets.

2 To use, melt a little of the oil in the palm of your hand and massage it into the hair and scalp.

3 Leave on for at least 2 hours and then shampoo off. Applying the shampoo to your hair before rinsing with water makes the oil easier to remove.

CARROT AND AVOCADO HAIR TREATMENT

This is a nourishing treatment for dry and neglected hair. Use jojoba oil as the base for the carrot macerate. These ingredients are sufficient for one treatment.

10 ml/2 tsp carrot macerated oil
1 ripe avocado

1 Prepare the macerated oil with grated carrot according to the recipe on page 22.

2 Mash the avocado, then blend it with the oil to make a paste.

3 Apply the mixture to the hair and scalp and leave for 1 hour.

4 Wash off, using a mild shampoo with added lemon juice.

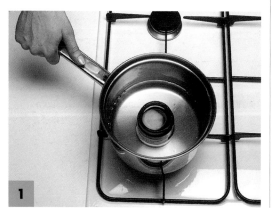
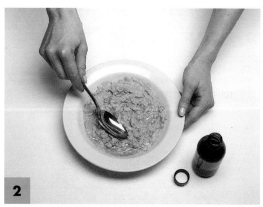

Conditioners

BANANA AND GRAPESEED
HAIR TREATMENT

A simple-to-make, deep conditioning treatment for dry hair. These ingredients are enough for one treatment.

1 ripe banana
10 ml/2 tsp grapeseed oil

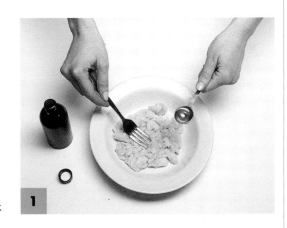

1 Mash the banana, using a fork, then mix with the oil to make a paste.

2 Massage into the hair and scalp, cover the hair with clingfilm (plastic wrap) and leave for 30 minutes.

3 Wash out, using a mild shampoo with added lemon juice.

QUICK TREATMENTS

❧ To treat dry hair, massage olive oil into the hair, paying particular attention to the ends if they are split, and wrap the hair in a warm towel. Leave for 1 hour and rinse out using a mild shampoo with added lemon juice.

❧ For a conditioning treatment, beat an egg and then rub it into the hair. Rinse out using an infusion of chamomile flowers. Use cool water, or the egg will set!

❧ Clay mixed with water to form a paste can be used instead of shampoo. Rhassoul is a special type of mud from Morocco, which is used specifically for this purpose.

❧ For extra shine and vitality, rub sweet almond oil into your scalp and hair. Leave in for 2 hours, then rub in natural yogurt and leave for a further 30 minutes. Wash out using a mild shampoo.

❧ If your hair is chlorine damaged, massage corn syrup into your scalp and hair. Leave for 30 minutes, and then wash out using a mild shampoo with added lemon juice.

Conditioners

CIDER VINEGAR TREATMENTS

Cider vinegar can be used to rinse and condition the hair and to restore the pH balance of the scalp. For extra effect, herbs such as rosemary, bay, sage and eucalyptus can be macerated in the vinegar. See the chart on page 31 for a guide to the use of herbs.

BEER RINSE FOR FINE HAIR

Beer is a traditional tonic for adding shine and body to fine hair. The smell of it fades when the hair dries. These ingredients are sufficient for one treatment.

1 pint beer
150 ml/¼ pt/⅔ cup cider vinegar

1 Blend the beer with the vinegar. Pour over your hair several times as the final rinse after shampooing, and then allow the hair to dry naturally.

APPLE AND THYME RINSE

A hair and scalp tonic, particularly good for treating dandruff. These ingredients are sufficient for one treatment.

10 drops wild thyme essential oil
100 ml/3½ fl oz/7 tbsp apple juice/apple cider vinegar

1 Blend the thyme essential oil with the apple juice or vinegar.

2 Massage the mixture into your scalp and leave for up to 5 minutes.

3 Rinse your hair with water and then shampoo it.

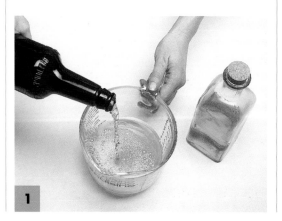

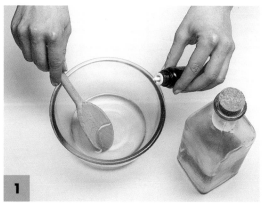

Hair Dyes and Highlighters

Before you use any natural hair dye, it is important to cover the skin around the hairline with ointment base to avoid any discoloration. When working out the length of time to leave the dye on the hair, the porosity of the hair and the colour required must be taken into consideration – the times given here are just a rough guide, and the effects are not guaranteed. Always condition the hair after applying colourant to rebalance the pH.

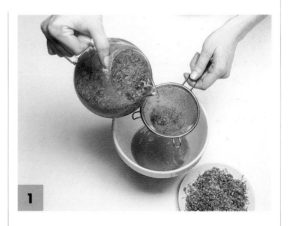

1

CHAMOMILE HIGHLIGHTER

For blonde hair. These ingredients are sufficient for one treatment.

**7 g/4 tbsp dried chamomile flowers
100 ml/3½ fl oz water**

1 Infuse the dried chamomile with water, allowing it to stand for 20 minutes before straining.

2 Apply to the hair, leave on for 20 minutes and rinse out.

INFUSIONS

Other herb infusions (see page 19) can be used as a final rinse after washing the hair. Rosemary will add shine and condition to dark hair; nettle will help alleviate dandruff or an itchy scalp. If you are using fresh herbs, they should be picked early in the day, before the sun is hot, because the heat of the sun causes any essential oil to evaporate from the leaves.

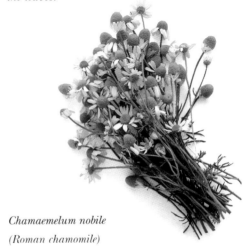

*Chamaemelum nobile
(Roman chamomile)*

Hair Dyes and Highlighters

WALNUT RINSE

For dark hair. These ingredients are sufficient
for one treatment.

100 ml/3½ fl oz water
2 tsp walnut leaves
1 teabag (black tea)

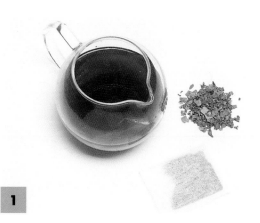

1 Decoct the water with walnut leaves and the tea bag. Allow to stand for 30 minutes.

1

2 Apply to the hair, leave for 30 minutes. Rinse out, then shampoo and condition the hair.

SAGE AND BLACK TEA

For grey hair. For the first couple of treatments
apply to the whole head. Thereafter, this
mixture can be used to touch up the roots every
couple of weeks. These ingredients are sufficient
for one treatment.

4 tbsp dried sage leaves
100 ml/3½ fl oz water
1 teabag (black tea)

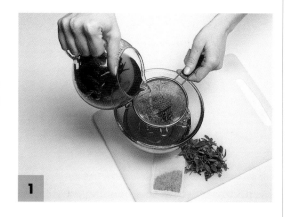

1

1 Decoct the water with the sage and teabag. Allow to stand for 30 minutes.

2 Apply to the hair, leave for 30 minutes. Rinse out, then shampoo and condition the hair.

Hair Dyes and Highlighters

Henna will colour the hair varying shades of red, depending on the country in which it was grown. Use hot water to make a paste with the powder and apply it, as hot as possible, to the hair, taking care to cover the roots. How long it should be left will depend on the freshness of the henna, your own hair and the heat of the water. Always test it on a small section of hair first to avoid unwanted results. Be careful not to stain your hands when you are using it, and remember that henna will stain bowls and washbasins, too.

HENNA RINSE

In the following recipe, tea will give a bright red; for a darker red, use coffee. These ingredients are sufficient for one treatment.

1 teabag (black tea) or 1 tsp ground coffee
100 g/3½ oz henna
15 ml/1 tbsp olive oil
250 ml/8 fl oz/1 cup water

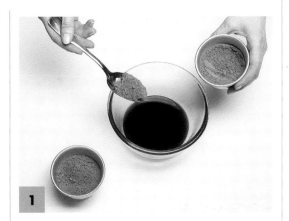

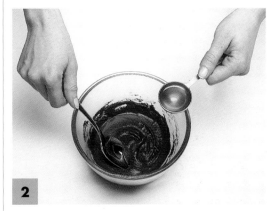

1 Make a cup of tea or coffee and add the henna.

2 Mix in the olive oil and add more water (if necessary) to make a smooth paste.

3 Apply immediately to the hair, then cover with clingfilm (plastic wrap), silver foil and a warm towel.

4 Leave on for 2–3 hours, then rinse, shampoo and condition the hair.

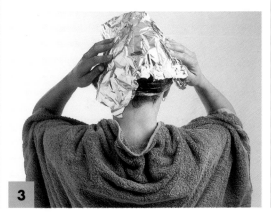

39

Special Treatments

STIMULATING HAIR OIL

This is a particularly useful treatment for hair loss. These ingredients are sufficient to make about 10 ml/2 tsp. It will keep for up to 12 months.

2 drops basil essential oil
2 drops rosemary essential oil
10 ml/2 tsp avocado oil

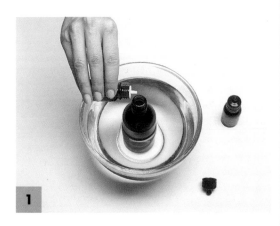

1 Mix the essential oils with the base oil (in this case avocado).

2 Heat the bottle before use in a bowl of hot water.

3 Massage the mixture into the scalp for at least 30 minutes. Repeat regularly for the best results.

ROSEMARY AND CEDARWOOD HAIR TREATMENT

The Neal's Yard Remedies Rosemary and Cedarwood Hair Treatment has received glowing praise in the past for helping hair to grow. It is very easy to make yourself. These ingredients are sufficient to make 100 g/3½ oz. The treatment will keep for up to 30 months.

100 g/3½ oz jar coconut oil
20 drops rosemary essential oil
10 drops cedarwood essential oil

1 Melt the coconut oil by standing the glass jar in a bowl of hot water.

2 Add the essential oils and mix thoroughly.

3 To use, warm some oil by rubbing it in the palm of your hand, and then methodically work it through your hair, concentrating on massaging the scalp.

4 Wrap a warm towel around your head and leave for 30 minutes.

5 Remove the oil by applying shampoo before adding water. Rinse and repeat if necessary.

Special Treatments

TREATMENT FOR HEAD LICE

This is a excellent treatment for lice. All bedding and clothes must also be washed to remove any eggs (see Head Lice Rinse). These ingredients are sufficient to make 100 ml/ 3½ fl oz. It will keep for up to 12 months.

20 drops geranium essential oil
20 drops lavender essential oil
20 drops rosemary essential oil
20 drops tea tree essential oil
100 ml/3½ fl oz/7 tbsp almond or coconut oil

1 Add the essential oils to the almond or coconut oil.

2 Depending on hair length, massage 10–15ml/2–3 tsp through the hair and all over the scalp. Cover the head and leave for 4 hours.

3 Massage the shampoo thoroughly through the hair before rinsing with water.

4 Comb the hair with a fine-toothed comb.

5 Repeat after 48 hours, and then again after 8 days.

HEAD LICE RINSE

You can replace the quassia used here with neem, a herb known for its insecticidal properties. However, it does not smell very inviting! These ingredients are sufficient for one treatment.

30 g/1 oz/5 tbsp quassia chips
600 ml/1 pt/2½ cups water

1 Either soak the quassia in water overnight or decoct it for 10 minutes.

2 Use this mix to wash down bedding, coat collars and so forth. It is also a good idea to use it as a weekly preventative hair rinse during a period of louse infestation at school.

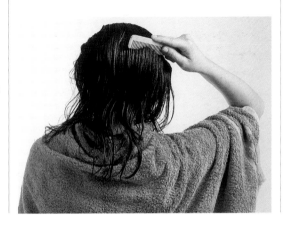

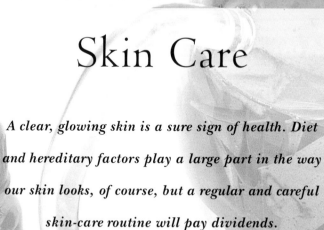

Skin Care

*A clear, glowing skin is a sure sign of health. Diet
and hereditary factors play a large part in the way
our skin looks, of course, but a regular and careful
skin-care routine will pay dividends.
The recipes here will cleanse, moisturize, tone and
otherwise pamper your skin, leaving it looking
smooth and youthful.*

The skin is one of the most amazing organs of the body – it has many physiological functions and at the same time provides us with information about the world as well as giving information about us to the world!

Much of the story our skin has to tell is about our inheritance. Hereditary factors determine much about our skin's colour, tendencies, type and susceptibility to certain skin problems. To some extent we can use this family history to forearm ourselves; if you know that your mother, for example, suffered from stretch marks or sun-damaged skin, and your skin type is basically similar, you can take special precautions.

Inheritance is not the whole story, though – diet and skin-care routine are also important factors in the appearance of the skin. The most important thing to remember is that the skin is alive; it is growing new cells and sloughing off old ones all the time, so changes are infinitely possible – for better and for worse. If you nurture your skin and look after it carefully with a regular skin-care regime, the results will be evident to all.

The physiological functions of the skin include getting rid of waste matter through the pores (elimination), protecting the body against foreign invaders such as bacteria, viruses and chemical pollutants, regulating body temperature, manufacturing vitamin D from sunlight and providing information about touch and pain. These functions mean that the skin is a good indicator of our general health – signs of prolonged stress or self-neglect will sooner or later show up on our skin. Remember, however, that even though a good skin-care routine and improving your diet and lifestyle can do much to transform tired, dingy or prematurely ageing skin, if you have a skin disease the best course of action is to see a natural health therapist who has experience of treating your type of skin condition.

THE STRUCTURE OF THE SKIN

The skin consists of two layers – an outer epidermis, where the process of continual skin renewal occurs, and an inner dermis. It is from

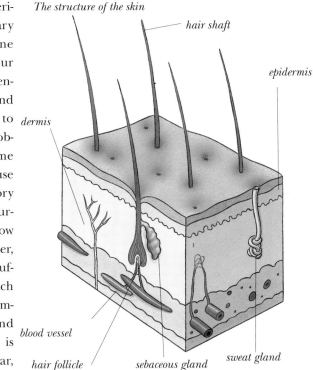

The structure of the skin

hair shaft

epidermis

dermis

blood vessel

hair follicle

sebaceous gland

sweat gland

the deepest region of the epidermis, the basal layer, that new cells are constantly produced. As the cells mature they are pushed closer to the surface by newer cells from below. While the cells migrate to the surface their nuclei are destroyed and replaced by a waterproofing protein called keratin. By the time they reach the *stratum corneum* (outer surface) the cells have been flattened, hardened, closely packed together and almost completely filled with keratin, forming a tough, protective and virtually waterproof layer.

The journey from basal layer to *stratum corneum* takes an estimated 14 days in young people (up to twice as long as we grow older), and approximately the same amount of time will elapse before the cells are sloughed off. In the region of 10 billion dead skin cells are sloughed off every 24 hours. In order for this process to work efficiently a fine balance between the production of new cells and the loss of old cells needs to be maintained.

Melanin-producing cells can be found interspersed throughout the basal layer. Melanin is the brown pigment that absorbs harmful ultra-violet rays from the sun and hence provides us with a natural protective screen. Exposure to the sun stimulates increased melanin production, and this results in the skin becoming darker – that is, it becomes tanned. When melanin is unable to absorb all the ultra-violet rays, because of prolonged and unaccustomed exposure, the skin is damaged and sunburn is experienced.

The inner, dermal layer is composed of connective tissue, containing both elastin – the fibres that give the qualities of stretch and suppleness to the skin – and collagen – the fibres that provide strength. The dermis is also infiltrated by numerous blood vessels.

Sweat glands provide the skin with its excretory function, ridding it of waste products, while also aiding in temperature regulation. Sweat glands can be divided into two types: eccrine glands and apocrine glands. Eccrine glands are distributed throughout the body but are found in higher densities on the soles of the feet and the palms of the hands. They secrete a watery fluid and are thought to react to adrenaline stimulation, which would explain why some people suffer from sweaty palms when they are nervous or anxious.

Apocrine glands occur in hairy parts of the body and only become active when puberty is reached. They are most notably found in the armpit and groin regions, and the distinctive odour associated with these areas is a result of the reaction between bacteria that naturally and harmlessly occupy the armpit and groin and the secretions from these glands.

Sebaceous glands are another type of gland found in the skin. These are larger on the face, scalp and shoulders. Sebaceous glands secrete an oily substance known as sebum, which keeps the skin and hair conditioned as well as providing antibacterial and antifungal protection.

THE AGEING PROCESS

The skin of small children is smooth, clear and glowing, but as the teenage years are reached evidence of hormonal activity begins to show on the skin, with the characteristic blackheads, acne and spots that can cause so much misery to the sufferer. With adolescence past, there is usually a period when we have youthful yet healthy looking skin with the minimum of effort.

From the age of about 25, our skin tends to become more dry as the levels of sebum drop. Then, from the age of about 50, the number of elastin fibres begins to decline radically and our skin starts to lose its natural elasticity and suppleness and the appearance of bags and sagging begins to accelerate. In addition to these ageing factors, the collagen fibres that are the underlying support structure of the skin become twisted and matted, causing wrinkles and lines.

The good news about collagen damage is that there are steps we can take to minimize it and even remedy damage already done. The main factors affecting collagen damage are exposure to ultra-violet light and free radical activity. This is the main reason why exposure to strong sunlight, and especially ultra-violet rays, can cause premature ageing. We can do much to avoid unnecessary damage to our skin by avoiding exposure to strong sunlight, using sunscreens and not using tanning beds.

Free radical activity can be reduced by the use of antioxidants. Externally, the most effective antioxidant is vitamin E and so it makes sense to use a night cream or moisturizer containing it (wheatgerm oil and avocado oil are good natural sources of vitamin E). Internally, antioxidants play a crucial part in our diet and slow down all the signs of ageing, including in the skin. Important antioxidants

in our diet are vitamins A, C and E, selenium and zinc, many of which are found in fresh fruit and vegetables. Other good things we can do to reduce the effects of ageing are to get plenty of fresh air and exercise, both of which help to oxygenate the cells of the body including the skin.

Smoking is one of the most damaging things you can do to your skin – it not only causes lines to appear around your mouth and blocks the skin's pores with irritating and toxic smoke particles, it also drastically accelerates the release of harmful free radicals. Alcohol can also tend to cause skin damage by exerting a drying effect and causing rapid dilation of the tiny capillaries in the dermis.

In general, the more you care for your skin and your overall health, the better you will be able to withstand the ravages of the ageing process. A good skin-care routine will pay dividends in years to come, even if it seems a bit of a chore at times. And even if you have left things until signs of neglect are beginning to appear, using a really good moisturizer and making improvements in your diet can still make a significant and visible difference.

KNOW YOUR SKIN TYPE

Knowing what skin type you have is important in helping you to choose which products are the most suitable and beneficial for you. Skin type can alter over time, and sometimes quite quickly; most people find, for example, that their skin becomes more liable to dryness as they get older. If you do find your skin type changing, be prepared to respond quickly with an adaptation of skin-care products.

DRY SKIN

Dry skin tends to be delicate and susceptible to flaking and fine lines. It can feel taut across the face, especially after cleansing. You should never use soap on dry skin; other things that exacerbate dryness are alcohol, exposure to the sun, central heating and wind. Gentle cleansing and careful moisturizing are a must. Herbs that are suitable for dry skin include chamomile, rose, comfrey, marsh mallow and marigold. Essential oils include chamomile, jasmine, neroli, palmarosa, rose and sandalwood.

NORMAL SKIN

Normal skin is soft, smooth, supple and not prone to eruptions. It should also have a healthy glow. Regular cleansing and the use of a light moisturizer are all that is needed to keep the skin looking clear and healthy. However, normal skin is often prone to becoming more dry as you grow older. Herbs suitable for normal skin include elderflower, marsh mallow, rose, marigold and lavender. Essential oils include geranium, lavender, palmarosa and rose.

OILY SKIN

Oily or greasy skin tends to be sallow and shiny and often has open pores. It is prone to blackheads and acne, but it does have the advantage of not wrinkling as easily as dry skin. Thorough yet gentle cleansing is a must for oily skin in order to keep the pores clear and reduce sebum build-up. The use of gentle astringent toners may also be helpful. Astringent herbs suitable for oily skin include elderflower, witch hazel, yarrow and lemon grass. Essential oils include cedarwood, cypress, vetiver, patchouli, orange and lemon.

COMBINATION SKIN

The face may have an oily section, usually a panel down the centre including the forehead, nose and chin, and areas of drier skin. You may find it best to treat the centre panel as oily skin and use different products for the drier areas, or use products that are balancing and recommended for normal skin. Balancing herbs include rose, lavender and elderflower. Essential oils include geranium, ylang ylang, bergamot and lavender.

PROBLEM SKIN

This is skin that is prone to blackheads (comedones), acne and spots. It is often oily, although not necessarily so. The most important factors here are diet, to help the skin with its eliminative process, and thorough yet gentle cleansing. If the acne is severe, consulting a professional therapist of natural medicine may be necessary to get the best results. Antiseptic and healing herbs include marigold, eucalyptus, yarrow, comfrey and elderflower. Essential oils include grapefruit, juniper, tea tree, lavender and bergamot. The use of clays for deep cleansing can also be very beneficial.

Sensitive skin

This type of skin is usually dry and prone to flaking, itching and redness. There may be a tendency to allergic reactions and also to broken capillaries. Exposure to strong sunlight and drinking alcohol will tend to make things worse. Cleansing should be a very gentle process and soothing and cooling moisturizers should be used. It is advisable to avoid the use of exfoliants, astringent toners and any products containing alcohol or fragrance. Soothing and anti-inflammatory herbs include chamomile, comfrey, marigold, chickweed and marsh mallow. Essential oils include chamomile, Roman chamomile, lavender and rose.

Mature skin

As the skin ages it loses elasticity and its ability to retain moisture and the signs of ageing appear, including sagging skin, fine lines and wrinkles. The emphasis of skin care is on nourishing and moisturizing the skin to reduce the effects of the ageing process. Regenerative herbs suitable for mature skin include rose, comfrey, marshmallow and marigold. Essential oils include olibanum, myrrh, rose, palmarosa, lavender and neroli.

CLEANSERS

The importance of cleansing to create and maintain healthy, clear, youthful and smooth skin cannot be over-emphasized. This is, of course, especially true if you wear make-up which, if left on the skin, will clog the pores and prevent it from breathing. Cleansing also removes dirt, excess sebum and the grime of pollution.

Cleansing should be a gentle as well as a thorough process, otherwise dryness or damage to delicate areas of skin can result. Soap can be very drying and should not really be used on the face. The simplest method of cleansing is to splash tepid water repeatedly over the face and then gently pat dry with a towel.

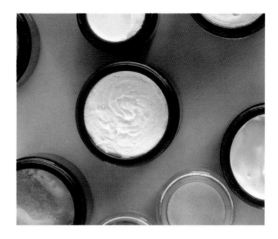

Many make-up products on the market today are water-resistant and designed to stay on for hours. This can make removing them difficult, but a basic and straightforward way of doing this is to pour a little olive oil or almond oil onto cotton wool and wipe the make-up off. Care should be taken around the eye area not to introduce any make-up into the eyes, as it may cause irritation. The use of a cleansing cream is one of the most effective techniques for removing make-up and for removing any dirt and grime that is trapped in the sebum on your skin. Cleansing creams are a combination of oil and water and help to loosen make-up and other dirt from the skin so that it can be wiped off with cotton wool.

To increase the efficiency of a cleanser, apply a face cloth soaked with warm water to the skin and allow it to sit there for a minute or so before cleansing. This will open the pores and soften the skin, thus enabling the cleanser to penetrate the skin and remove dirt more effectively. Then pour cleanser onto cotton wool and apply it to the face and neck, paying particular attention to the hairline, which is a common area for dirt and debris to build up. Areas of higher sebum secretion, such as the nose and chin, may also require extra care. Remember to choose a cleanser that is suitable for your skin type; if your skin feels taut after using a cleanser, it may be too drying for you.

Once the make-up and grime are off your skin, you can take the opportunity to massage your face to increase the blood flow to the skin and soften it in preparation for other treatments.

As well as daily cleansing of make-up and dirt it is a real treat for your skin to have an occasional deep-cleansing treatment such as a facial steam or a face pack. If you have oily or problem skin this can be done every couple of days; once a week should be often enough for normal or dry skin. Exfoliating (removing dead skin cells) can also spruce up tired or dingy-looking skin and there are plenty of natural ways to do this, the simplest of which is gently rubbing the skin with a 100 per cent cotton face cloth. However, exfoliation is not to be recommended for very sensitive skin.

The chart below is a guide to the essential oils and herbal infusions that are recommended for specific skin types. Use this information when you are creating your own skin preparations.

SKIN TYPE	ESSENTIAL OILS	HERBAL INFUSIONS
DRY	Chamomile, neroli, palmarosa, rose, sandalwood	Comfrey, chamomile, marigold, marsh mallow, rose
NORMAL	Geranium, lavender, palmarosa, rose	Elderflower, marigold, marsh mallow, rose
OILY	Cedarwood, cypress, lemon, orange, patchouli, vetiver	Elderflower, lemon grass, witch hazel, yarrow
COMBINATION	Bergamot, geranium, lavender, ylang ylang	Elderflower, lavender, rose
PROBLEM	Bergamot, grapefruit, juniper, lavender, tea tree	Comfrey, elderflower, eucalyptus, marigold, yarrow
SENSITIVE	Chamomile, lavender, Roman chamomile, rose	Chamomile, chickweed, comfrey, marsh mallow
MATURE	Lavender, myrrh, neroli, olibanum, palmarosa, rose	Comfrey, marigold, marsh mallow, rose

Cleansers

WASHING BALL

A washing ball is an unusual idea, resembling a small ball of dough. It has a gritty consistency, which is very different from the smooth lather we are used to from soap. However, it does cleanse the face without dehydrating the skin, and regular use will result in a smooth complexion.

125 g/4 oz/5 tbsp raisins
125 g/4 oz/15 tbsp ground almonds
2 slices soft brown bread

1 Depending on the size, finely chop the raisins. Mix the almonds with the raisins.

2 Finely crumble the bread and add to the mixture. Alternatively, use a blender to mix all of the above ingredients.

3 Roll the mixture into between six and ten balls and use instead of soap.

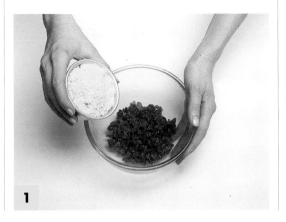

1

FACIAL STEAMS

Steaming the face is an excellent way of deep-cleansing the skin. The steam opens the pores of the skin, allowing the active constituents of the herbs and oils used to be really effective. **Note:** Facial steams are not recommended if you have thread veins or very delicate skin.

METHOD

Either fill a bowl with boiling water and add the required essential oils or pour boiling water over a handful of herbs. Place a towel over your head and the bowl and remain there for 5 minutes. Do be careful, though, not to persist if you are finding it uncomfortable. Too much heat can be damaging, as can breathing in the oils if you find them overpowering – so be gentle! Only add 1 drop of oil in a bowl of water until you become confident that the effects are beneficial. Remember to close the pores after this cleansing process by using an astringent toner.

SIMPLE CLEANSING SUGGESTIONS

* The Cream Base on page 24 can be used instead of soap.

* Plain live yogurt can be used as a cleanser. Apply with cotton wool to remove dirt before toning and moisturizing the face. This is particularly good for problem skin.

* Sweet almond oil can be used to take off all make-up including eye make-up.

Face Packs and Masks

These face packs are made using fresh fruit and are therefore quite messy, so make sure you have plenty of towels ready to protect your clothes. All these recipes are sufficient for one treatment.

APPLE AND CINNAMON FACE PACK

An antiseptic mask for oily or problem skin.

1 ripe apple, peeled and grated
½ tsp single (light) cream
1 tsp clear honey
1 tbsp ground oats
½ tsp ground cinnamon

1 Combine all the ingredients in a bowl and mash into a paste, using a fork.

2 Apply the pack to your face and leave on for 10 minutes. Gently remove with cool water, then pat dry with a clean towel.

BANANA FACE PACK

A rich and nourishing face pack for dry skin.

1 egg yolk
10 ml/2 tsp almond oil
1 ripe banana

1 Combine all the ingredients in a bowl and mash into a paste, using a fork.

2 Apply the pack to your face and leave on for 10 minutes. Gently remove with cool water, then pat dry with a clean towel.

AVOCADO AND HONEY FACE PACK

A nourishing and regenerating facial for rejuvenating tired or mature skin.

1 ripe avocado
5 ml/1 tsp clear honey
5 ml/1 tsp lemon juice
5 ml/1 tsp plain yogurt

1 Combine all the ingredients in a bowl and mash into a paste, using a fork. Leave in the refrigerator for 30 minutes.

2 Apply the pack to your face and leave on for 10 minutes. Gently remove with cool water, then pat dry with a clean towel.

GRAPEFRUIT MASK

A skin-toning facial treatment, naturally rich in AHAs (alpha hydroxy acids), suitable for all skin types.

1 grapefruit
1 small pot plain yogurt

1 Peel the grapefruit, break the flesh into segments and remove the seeds and pith.

2 Blend enough yogurt with the fruit to make a paste. Leave the mixture for 1 hour in the refrigerator.

3 Apply the pack to your face and leave on for 10 minutes. Gently remove with cool water, then pat dry with a clean towel.

Face Packs and Masks

STRAWBERRY AND OAT EXFOLIATING MASK

A gentle exfoliating face pack to cleanse and tone the skin. These ingredients are sufficient for one treatment.

20 g/2 tbsp ground oats
3 large ripe strawberries
5 ml/1 tsp single (light) cream

1 Grind the oats to a fine powder, using a mortar and pestle or blender.

2 Mash up the strawberries, using a fork, and mix with the oats. Add enough cream to make a paste.

3 Apply the pack to your face and leave on for 10 minutes.

4 Gently remove with cool water, then pat dry with a clean towel.

LAVENDER AND WITCH HAZEL MASK

This face mask unblocks and tightens pores and absorbs excess sebum. These ingredients are sufficient for one treatment.

2 tsp fuller's earth
2 tsp witch hazel
1 egg, lightly beaten
2 drops lavender essential oil

1 Mix the fuller's earth with the witch hazel to make a paste.

2 Add the beaten egg and mix in the essential oil.

3 Apply the pack to your face and leave on for 10 minutes.

4 Gently remove with cool water, then pat dry with a clean towel.

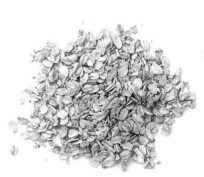
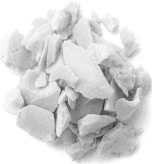

Face Packs and Masks

CLAY MASK 1

This is suitable for most skin types, except very dry skin. The ingredients are sufficient for one or two treatments. It will keep for 3 months.

30 ml/2 tbsp aloe vera
5 ml/1 tsp witch hazel
5 ml/1 tsp clear honey
½ tbsp kaolin
1 tbsp bentonite
1 drop lavender essential oil

1 Mix together the aloe vera, witch hazel and honey.

2 To this mixture, slowly add the kaolin and bentonite, stirring constantly. Force the mixture through a sieve (strainer). Add the essential oil and mix in thoroughly.

3 Gently apply the mask over the face, avoiding the eyes. Leave on for 10 minutes, then wash off with warm water.

VARIATIONS

Flower waters may be substituted for the witch hazel in either mask, according to your skin type:

Problem skin: Lavender flower water

Oily skin: Witch hazel

Mature skin: Rosewater

Normal skin: Orange flower water

CLAY MASK 2

Try this slightly different recipe if you have more oily skin, or suffer from blackheads. These ingredients are sufficient for one or two treatments. It will keep for 3 months.

30 ml/2 tbsp aloe vera
5 ml/1 tsp witch hazel
5 ml/1 tsp fresh grapefruit juice
1½ tbsp kaolin
½ tbsp bentonite
1 drop lemon essential oil

1 Mix together the aloe vera, witch hazel and grapefruit juice.

2 Slowly add the kaolin and bentonite, stirring. Force the mixture through a sieve (strainer). Add the essential oil and mix.

3 Gently apply the mask over the face, avoiding the eyes. Leave on for 10 minutes, then wash off with warm water.

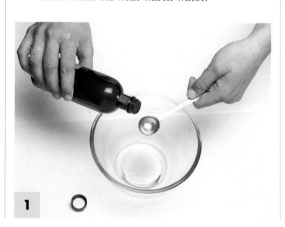

1

Toners

Toners are used to cool and refresh the skin. They also remove any remaining traces of dirt and any oiliness left from your cleanser. They are useful for oily skin, as many of them are astringent and help to reduce sebum levels and refine open pores.

In former times toners were often flower waters such as rosewater or lavender water, the by-product of essential oil distillation. These days flower waters are often manufactured by mixing essential oil with water, using a dispersant. Many skin toners contain a small amount of alcohol, which is fine if you have oily skin but may be rather drying for very dry or sensitive skin.

INFUSIONS AS TONERS

Many herbal infusions can be used as skin toners when cooled. See the chart on page 48 to find the right herb for your skin type.

LAVENDER AND WITCH HAZEL

Make a lavender and witch hazel infusion. The antiseptic and astringent properties make it particularly appropriate for oily or problem skin.

PARSLEY WATER

Soak fresh parsley (use organic if possible) in still mineral water overnight. This parsley water can be used to tone the skin and is particularly good for cleansing the skin of blackheads.

LEMON AND GLYCERINE

This mixture has a slightly astringent and strengthening effect on the capillaries; use it if you have thread veins. These ingredients will make 20 ml/3 tsp. It will keep for 3 months.

**20 ml/4 tsp vegetable glycerine
juice of 1 lemon
1 drop neroli essential oil
1 drop rose absolute**

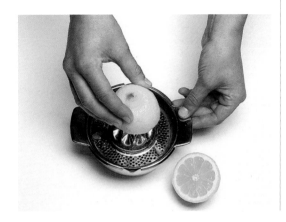

1 Mix the vegetable glycerine with the lemon juice and add the essential oils.

2 Apply twice a day to thread veins.

Toners

REFRESHING SPRITZER

This is a beneficial face or body spray. These ingredients are sufficient to make 100 ml/3½ fl oz. Keep it in the refrigerator when not in use and replace every 2 days.

2 heaped tsp fresh mint
2 heaped tsp fresh dill
1 heaped tsp fresh parsley
85 ml/3 fl oz/⅓ cup mineral water

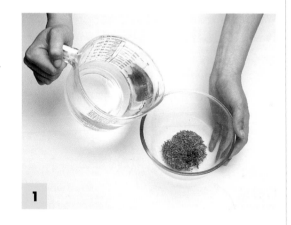

1 Using the herbs above, make a strong infusion (see page 19).

2 Add the mineral water to the infusion and pour the mixture into a bottle with an atomizer attachment.

REFRESHING FACE SPRAY

A spray that is particularly good for dry skin. If your skin tends to be greasy, use witch hazel instead of orange flower water. These ingredients are sufficient to make 100 ml/3½ fl oz. It will keep for up to 2 days in the refrigerator.

85 ml/3 fl oz/⅓ cup distilled water
10 ml/2 tsp aloe vera
2 ml/½ tsp orange flower water
1 drop propolis tincture
1 drop neroli essential oil
1 drop rosemary essential oil

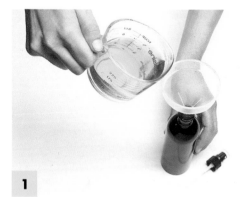

1 Combine the ingredients and store in a bottle. Shake before using with an atomizer spray.

54

Moisturizers

Moisturizers are probably the most popular cosmetic product, and they are certainly a very important part of any skin-care routine. A good moisturizer should rehydrate the skin and keep it feeling supple without making it feel greasy or preventing the skin from being able to breathe. It can also help to protect the skin by providing a barrier against pollutants and irritants, and the latest generation of moisturizers often have a sunscreen added to protect the skin from the harmful effects of the sun.

Moisturizers need to combine an oil for emollient properties, which help to keep the skin supple, and water for moisturizing, rehydrating properties. In order to keep the oil and water combined an emulsifier will be needed. The simplest emulsifiers are beeswax and borax, and we use these in the following recipes.

Because moisturizers are formulated to penetrate the surface of the skin, they are the ideal way to deliver therapeutic ingredients to it. This is true whether they are made of highly technological ingredients or natural ingredients such as herbs and essential oils.

RESTORING PH

If your skin has been dehydrated by using soap, you can restore the pH balance by splashing your face daily with 5 ml/1 tsp cider vinegar diluted in 600 ml/1 pint/2½ cups water. You could make an extraction of elderflowers in the vinegar for an extra cleansing effect.

LAVENDER AND LEMON MOISTURIZER

A moisturizer with antiseptic and healing properties suitable for oily or problem skin. This recipe makes a 40 g/1½ oz jar.

1 tsp beeswax (granules or grated)
5 g cocoa butter
45 ml/3 tbsp grapeseed oil
½ tsp borax
30 ml/1 fl oz/2 tbsp lavender infusion
10 drops lemon essential oil

1 Heat the beeswax, cocoa butter and base oil in a bowl over a saucepan of boiling water.

2 Dissolve the borax in the lavender infusion.

3 Slowly add the infusion to the oil mixture, stirring constantly.

4 When the mixture cools down, add the essential oil.

5 Store in a dark glass jar in the refrigerator. It will keep for up to 2 months.

Moisturizers

AVOCADO MOISTURIZER

A rich and nourishing moisturizer for dry skin.
This recipe makes a 40 g/1½ oz jar.

1 tsp beeswax (granules or grated)
5 g cocoa butter
15 ml/1 tbsp avocado oil
30 ml/1 fl oz/2 tbsp almond oil
½ tsp borax
30 ml/1 fl oz/2 tbsp marsh mallow infusion
5 drops sandalwood essential oil
5 drops bergamot essential oil

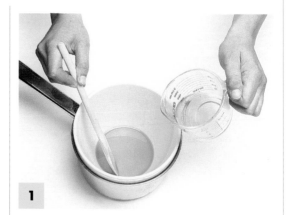

1 Heat the beeswax, cocoa butter and base oils in a bowl set over a saucepan of boiling water.

2 Dissolve the borax in the marsh mallow infusion.

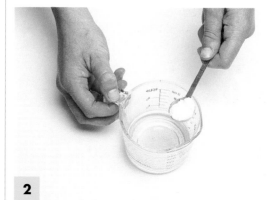

3 Slowly add the infusion to the oil mixture, stirring constantly.

4 When the mixture cools down, add the essential oils.

5 Store in a dark glass jar in the refrigerator. It will keep for up to 2 months.

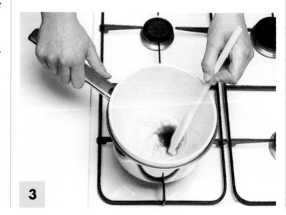

Moisturizers

GERANIUM AND APRICOT MOISTURIZER

A light and balancing moisturizer for normal or combination skin. This recipe makes a 40 g/1½ oz jar.

1 tsp beeswax (granules or grated)
5 g cocoa butter
15 ml/½ fl oz/1 tbsp apricot kernel oil
30 ml/1 fl oz/2 tbsp grapeseed oil
½ tsp borax
2 tbsp rose petal infusion
10 drops geranium essential oil

1 Heat the beeswax, cocoa butter and base oils in a bowl set over a saucepan of boiling water.

2 Dissolve the borax in the rose petal infusion. Slowly add the infusion to the oil mixture, stirring constantly.

3 When the mixture cools down, add the essential oil.

4 Store in a dark glass jar in the refrigerator. It will keep for up to 2 months.

ROSE FACIAL OIL

This is an exquisite oil suitable for delicate skin. Apply nightly for a luxurious and rejuvenating facial massage. It also makes a delightful conditioning oil when applied to damp skin. This recipe makes a 30 ml/1 fl oz bottle.

10 ml/2 tsp evening primrose oil
20 ml/4 tsp grapeseed oil
5 drops rose absolute
5 drops patchouli essential oil
5 drops geranium essential oil

1 Blend the base oils and essential oils together.

2 Store in a dark glass bottle. It will last for up to 6 months.

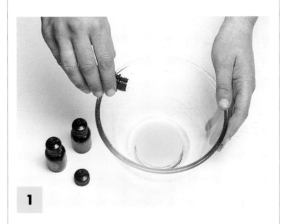

1

Measure small amounts of liquid with a dropper – 20 drops is approximately 1 ml.

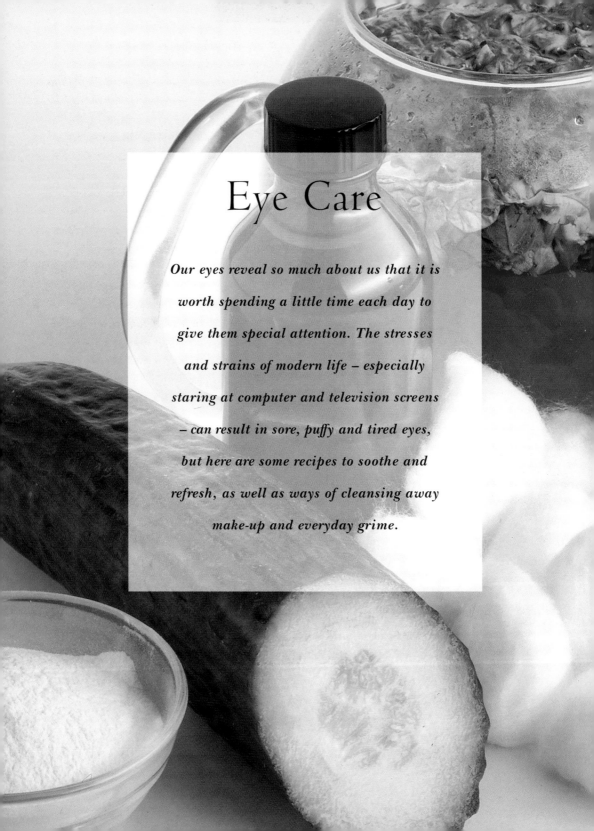

Eye Care

*Our eyes reveal so much about us that it is
worth spending a little time each day to
give them special attention. The stresses
and strains of modern life – especially
staring at computer and television screens
– can result in sore, puffy and tired eyes,
but here are some recipes to soothe and
refresh, as well as ways of cleansing away
make-up and everyday grime.*

We tend to take our eyes for granted, although they are one of the most vital of our organs. They deserve to be looked after for they convey much of who and how we are to the world around us.

The best recipe for the eyes is of course to look after your general health. Remember, too, that eyes need rest. With the increasing use of computer screens at work and television at home, eyes are subject to extra strain which can result in puffiness and soreness. Exercise can help to alleviate puffiness, while sleep and a balanced diet of fresh and whole foods will be good for your eyes and for your general well-being. Drink lots of water and avoid salt, caffeine and alcohol.

Tired or strained eyes can be soothed by being bathed in herbal infusions. Chamomile is often used, but even more effective is an infusion made with the leaves of *Euphrasia officinalis*, commonly known as eyebright. The astringent and anti-inflammatory properties of this herb have made it a traditional treatment for eye irritations, including conjunctivitis and the soreness caused by fatigue or being in a smoky atmosphere. In another traditional recipe for eye infections, eyebright is combined with golden seal (*Hydrastis canadensis*) to make a soothing eye bath.

The skin around the eyes is especially delicate. Always take great care when you are removing eye make-up. A little almond oil on cotton wool will quickly remove most make-up, or try the Eye Make-up Remover cream on page 61.

Whenever you make and use any preparations for your eyes, be especially scrupulous about sterilizing the equipment you use. Eye infections can be very quickly transmitted and cleanliness at all times is absolutely essential.

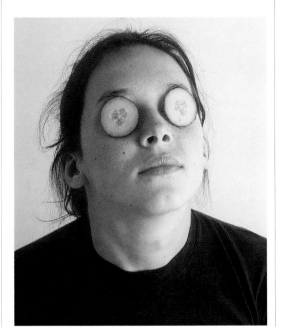

RELIEVING TIRED EYES

If your eyes feel tired or have bags under them try lying back, closing your eyes and applying one of the following

* Dry, sore eyes: cotton wool pads soaked in aloe vera juice

* Hot, sore eyes: slices of cooling cucumber

* Puffy eyes: slices of potato

* Tired eyes: used chamomile teabags (preferably organic); other herbs that will help include witch hazel, calendula and elderflower

Refreshers

EYE BATHS

Eyes can benefit from bathing, but make sure your hands are washed and that any equipment you use is free from dirt or contamination.

1 Prepare a herbal infusion (see page 19) with the appropriate herbs (see below). Herbal infusions must be made fresh daily.

2 Strain through muslin (cheesecloth) or an unbleached coffee filter to ensure that no irritating herb particles are present.

3 Use an eye bath or an eggcup that has been sterilized with boiling water. Tip your head back, holding the eye bath to your eye.

4 Clean the eye bath in between bathing each eye to avoid spreading any infection.

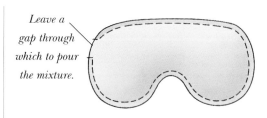

Leave a gap through which to pour the mixture.

EYE BAGS

Eye bags look and feel rather like eyemask-shaped beanbags and it is a simple sewing job to make them up. The linseed is very cooling to the skin, a property that cotton wool does not have, and it will absorb the essential oils.

100 g/3½ oz/5 tbsp linseeds
2 drops neroli essential oil
2 drops lavender essential oil

1 Choose some very soft fabric that you feel would be comfortable placed over your eyes. A close-weave cotton such as lawn is probably best. Cut out two shapes (see diagram) that will cover both eyes.

2 Stitch together all the way around the edges, leaving a small gap through which you pour the linseed to which a mixture of 2 drops each of neroli and lavender essential oils have been added. Close up the gap.

3 Lie down, place the bags over your eyes and relax. When the fragrance has faded, just open up the bag and add some more drops of essential oils.

HERBS FOR EYE BATHS

❀ Tired eyes: rose petals

❀ Strained eyes: eyebright and chamomile

❀ Conjunctivitis: eyebright and marigold

Gels and Lotions

EYE GEL

This is a wonderful gel to help tighten the skin around the eyes and reduce puffiness. Great care must be taken when using products around the eyes. Do not put this cooling and toning gel into the eyes, or where it can seep in. These ingredients will make 65 ml/4 tbsp. Store in the refrigerator and do not use longer than a week after making it.

20 ml/4 tsp cornflower infusion
20 ml/4 tsp calendula infusion
1 g/¼ tsp carrageen
20 ml/4 tsp distilled water
5 ml/1 tsp euphrasia tincture

1 Make the cornflower and calendula infusions as directed on page 19.

2 Mix the carrageen with the distilled water until fully dissolved.

3 Add the infusions to the distilled water along with the tincture and allow to set.

EYE MAKE-UP REMOVER

To remove make-up, gently wipe the eyes with a little almond oil on cotton wool. Alternatively, try the following cream, which uses chamomile infusion to soothe. The ingredients given here will make approximately 100 ml/3 fl oz.

1 tsp beeswax (granules or grated)
½ tsp shea nut butter
¼ tsp cocoa butter
10 ml/2 tsp almond oil
2 ml/40 drops aloe vera juice
70 ml/14 tsp chamomile infusion
10 ml/2 tsp cetyl stearyl alcohol

1 Heat the beeswax, shea nut butter, cocoa butter and almond oil together until melted.

2 Add the aloe vera juice to the chamomile infusion. Mix in the alcohol which is available from pharmacies. Heat the mixture.

3 Check the temperatures of the oil mix and the infusion mix. When both are 70°C/158°F, mix them together with a hand whisk.

4 Allow to cool before pouring into a dark-coloured glass bottle. The cream will keep for up to 3 weeks in the refrigerator.

Mouth and Ear Care

*After our eyes, people tend to notice our
mouths. Smooth lips and gleaming teeth
will make a friendly smile doubly
welcoming, and the confidence that comes
from the certainty that our breath is fresh
and sweet will affect our whole demeanour.
Use natural ingredients in your daily
routines, and notice the difference.*

Toothpastes and Mouthwashes

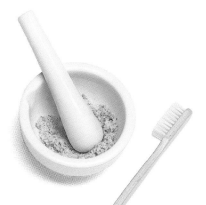

LAVENDER AND LEMON MOUTHWASH

An antiseptic and healing mouthwash for sore gums that will also freshen the breath. These ingredients are sufficient to make 90 ml/3 fl oz/ 6 tbsp. It will keep for up to 6 months.

15 ml/3 tsp lavender tincture
15 ml/3 tsp calendula tincture
50 ml/10 tsp vegetable glycerine
2 drops lemon essential oil
2 drops orange essential oil
5 drops peppermint essential oil

1 Blend all the ingredients together and pour them into a bottle.

2 Shake the bottle and dilute 1 teaspoon in a little water to rinse around the mouth.

VARIATIONS
If the gums are bleeding, try adding raspberry tincture. Echinacea, myrrh or golden seal tinctures are good for infections. (In each case replace the lavender tincture.)

PEPPERMINT TOOTHPASTE

A simple toothpaste for regular use. Fennel or lemon essential oil can be used instead of peppermint if you prefer. If your teeth are aching add clove, which will help anaesthetize the pain. These ingredients are sufficient for one treatment.

1 tsp sodium bicarbonate
5 ml/1 tsp vegetable glycerine
3 drops peppermint essential oil

1 Mix the sodium bicarbonate with the vegetable glycerine.

2 Add the essential oil.

SAGE AND MYRRH TOOTHPOWDER

An excellent remedy for sore and bleeding gums. These ingredients are sufficient for one treatment.

1 g/½ tbsp sage
5 g/1 tsp salt
5 drops myrrh essential oil

1 Grind the sage and salt together, using a mortar and pestle.

2 Add the essential oil, preferably spraying through an atomizer.

3 Brush on to your teeth and gums, using a toothbrush. Do not swallow.

Lip Balms

MANDARIN LIP BALM

The balm will keep for up to 6 months.

5 g/1 tsp beeswax
70 g/2¾ oz cocoa butter
1 tsp coconut oil
5 drops St John's wort tincture
5 drops calendula tincture
10 drops mandarin essential oil

1 Melt the beeswax, cocoa butter and coconut oil in a bowl over a saucepan of hot water.

2 Add the tinctures and then the essential oils.

3 Pour into a jar before the mixture begins to harden.

GRAPEFRUIT CONDITIONING LIP BALM

A moisturizing and naturally antiseptic lip balm for dry or sore lips. It will keep for up to 6 months.

1 g cocoa butter
9 g shea or cocoa butter
10 drops grapefruit essential oil

1 Melt the cocoa and shea butter over a bowl of hot water.

2 Add the essential oil and pour into jars. Leave to set. This may take up to 12 hours, depending on room temperature.

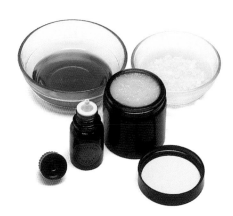

MOISTURIZING HERBAL LIP BALM

In this recipe, almond oil has been used to moisturize and hydrate the delicate skin of the lips; wheatgerm oil is high in vitamin E, which is an antioxidant and acts as a natural preservative; carrot oil is high in vitamin C; and myrrh essential oil is good for dry and chapped skin.

20 g/1½ tbsp beeswax (granules or grated)
50 ml/10 tsp almond oil
14 ml/scant 3 tsp wheatgerm oil
5 ml/1 tsp carrot oil
2 drops lemon essential oil
1 drop myrrh essential oil

1 Put the beeswax, almond, wheatgerm and carrot oils into a saucepan and heat slowly. Stir the mixture until all the beeswax has melted.

2 Remove the mixture from the heat and allow to cool slightly. Add the essential oils, pour the mixture into a container and allow to set.

Special Treatments

EARACHE

The following will help to relieve earache, but do seek professional assistance if the pain is extreme or persistent.

Garlic macerate or mullein macerate (see page 23) can be used, putting a few drops of the warm oil onto a piece of cotton wool and placing gently inside the ear. Remember not to put anything into the ear that is not clean – nor, as the old saying goes, anything smaller than your elbow. Do not put anything into your ear if your eardrum is perforated.

EAR/BODY PIERCING

There are a number of antibacterial and antiseptic herbs and oils that can be used after piercing. Make an infusion from echinacea or golden seal, and dab on to prevent infection. Alternatively, dab on a drop of lavender or tea tree essential oil.

TOOTHACHE

Apply clove essential oil to a cottonwool bud and hold on to the tooth. Teething pain can be soothed by rubbing the gums with marsh-mallow root decoction, or by allowing the baby to chew on a piece of orris or marsh mallow root. Teething problems can be relieved by giving Chamomilla granules 6X (a homeopathic remedy) as required.

COLD SORES

Apply tea tree essential oil to the skin at the first sign of a cold sore developing. Continue to use until the cold sore has dried up. Dab on calendula tincture to dry up and heal a cold sore. For the last stage of the cold sore, apply calendula ointment.

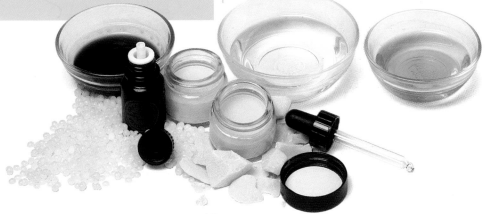

Hand Care

Tending our hands and nails should be part of our daily routine. Our hands, often unprotected, are plunged in and out of water; we garden and wash up without wearing gloves; we expose our hands to the wind and sun – and the neglect becomes only too evident as we age. Use these recipes to soften and protect your hands, and pay particular attention to your nails with some special conditioners and strengtheners.

Hand Creams

Many people do not realize until too late that the hands can give away the age quicker than a carefully protected face. A little time spent in putting on hand cream and taking care to wear gloves when washing up or gardening will make a great difference.

For centuries, women have been creating hand creams and using skin whiteners to conceal age spots and loose skin. Here are a few recipes for hand care that are fun to make and wonderful to use.

CHAMOMILE AND OAT
MOISTURIZING HAND SCRUB

A good alternative to soap for sensitive hands. These ingredients are sufficient to make 40 g/1½ oz.

30 ml/2 tbsp vegetable glycerine
15 g/½ oz/2 tbsp cornflour (cornstarch)
5 ml/1 tsp chamomile flower water
2 tsp finely ground oats
2 tsp finely ground rice

1 Heat the vegetable glycerine over a bowl of hot water.

2 Slowly add the cornflour (cornstarch), stirring constantly to make a paste.

3 Take off the heat and slowly add the chamomile water, still stirring. Stir in the ground oats and ground rice.

4 Store in a jar and use in the same way as liquid soap. It will keep for up to 2 months.

ROSE AND ALMOND HAND CREAM

This is a wonderful, rich hand cream. An infusion of chamomile or elderflower can be substituted for the rosewater. The recipe makes two 40 g/1½ oz jars.

8 g/1½ tsp cocoa butter
5 g/1 tsp beeswax (granules or grated)
30 ml/2 tbsp almond oil
45 ml/3 tbsp rosewater
½ tsp borax
10 drops rose absolute

1 Melt the cocoa butter, beeswax and almond oil over a bowl of hot water.

2 Heat the rosewater slightly and dissolve the borax into it.

3 Stir the rosewater and borax into the oily mixture very slowly and stir until the cream cools.

4 Add the rose absolute and stir. Store in a jar in the refrigerator. It will keep for up to 2 months.

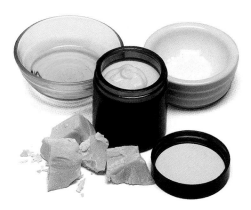

Hand Creams

ORANGE AND OLIBANUM HAND CREAM

*This is another rich cream, suitable
for dry, work-worn hands.
The recipe makes two 40 g/1½ oz jars.*

8 g/1½ tsp cocoa butter
5 g/1 tsp beeswax (granules or grated)
**10 ml/2 tsp almond oil and
wheatgerm oil, mixed**
45 ml/1½ fl oz/3 tbsp orange flower water
½ tsp borax
10 drops orange essential oil
5 drops olibanum essential oil

1 Melt the cocoa butter, beeswax and almond and wheatgerm oil over a bowl of hot water.

2 Heat the orange flower water slightly and dissolve the borax into it.

3 Stir the orange flower water and borax into the oily mixture very slowly.

4 Stir until the cream cools. Add the essential oils and stir.

5 Store in a jar in the refrigerator. It will keep for up to 2 months.

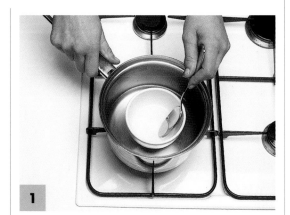

1

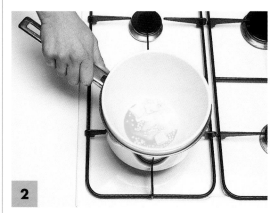

2

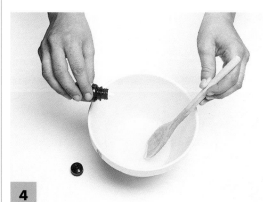

4

Nail Treatments

CUTICLE HARDENER

Squeeze the juice of half a lemon into a bowl of hot water and soak your hands for a few minutes. Repeat daily.

AYURVEDIC NAIL FORMULA

To condition and strengthen the nails.

15 ml/½ fl oz/1 tbsp almond oil
2 drops sandalwood essential oil
2 drops cypress essential oil
2 drops lavender essential oil

1 Blend all the oils together and store in a bottle.

2 To use, heat the bottle of blended oils in a bowl of hot water.

3 Apply daily to the nails on cotton wool buds. It will keep for up to 6 months.

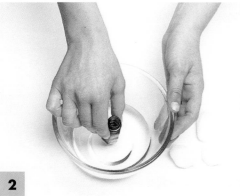

MYRRH NAIL STRENGTHENER

Use this nail strengthener daily. The ingredients are sufficient for one treatment.

25 ml/1½ tbsp horsetail infusion
15 g/1 tbsp lanolin
10 drops myrrh

1 Hold the nails in a bowl containing the horsetail infusion and leave for at least 5 minutes.

2 Mix together the lanolin and myrrh and rub thoroughly into the nails. Wash off any excess.

LEMON CUTICLE CONDITIONER

1 g cocoa butter
9 g/1½ tsp shea butter
10 drops lemon essential oil

1 Melt the cocoa butter and shea butter together in a bowl set over hot water.

2 Stir in the essential oil.

3 Pour the mixture into jars and leave to set – this may take up to 12 hours, depending on room temperature. It will keep for up to 3 months.

2

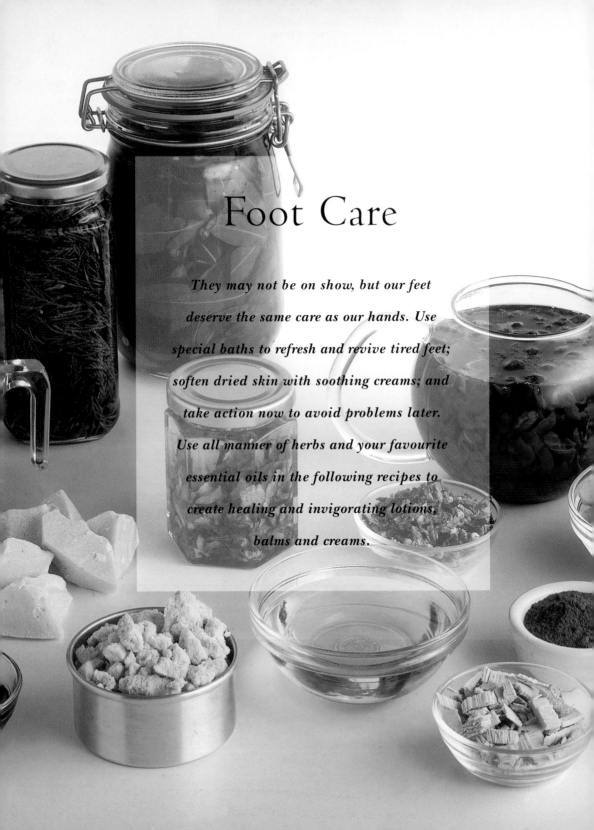

Foot Care

They may not be on show, but our feet

deserve the same care as our hands. Use

special baths to refresh and revive tired feet;

soften dried skin with soothing creams; and

take action now to avoid problems later.

Use all manner of herbs and your favourite

essential oils in the following recipes to

create healing and invigorating lotions,

balms and creams.

A lot of us complain about our feet killing us, but we expect them to put up with us walking for miles in shoes that are often badly suited to them – then we try to ignore any problems, hoping they will just go away.

Give your feet a treat and prepare a foot bath, for there's nothing better than soaking tired and aching feet when you get home after a long day – a washing up bowl half full of warm water is easy enough to arrange. Dead Sea Salts or sea salt are refreshing and cleansing. Add infused herbs such as marsh mallow, witch hazel, rosemary, thyme, comfrey and calendula; also choose from essential oils of lavender, eucalpytus, tea tree, rosemary, peppermint, geranium, thyme, tagetes. Use tincture of arnica for bruised and aching feet, while Epsom salts will help revive them.

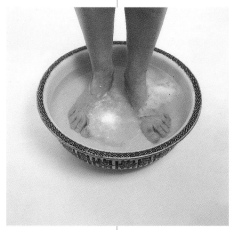

With 250,000 sweat glands covering the soles of the feet it is no wonder that they may feel a little on the damp side from time to time! The distinctive odour often associated with the feet results from the reaction between bacteria (naturally and harmlessly found in this area) and sweat. Washing the feet with soap and wearing cotton socks to reduce sweating will help, as will some of the suggestions in this section, especially the Lavender and Lemon Foot Deodorant and the Blackcurrant and Lemon Foot Powder on page 76. They have all been tried with varying results!

Corns develop due to repeated pressure and trauma, commonly forming either between or over the joints of the toes. To alleviate them, soak your feet in a bowl of warm water with 6–8 drops of tagetes essential oil added. Remove the build-up of hard skin using myrrh and mandarin foot scrub, or use a pumice stone directly on the corn.

Athlete's foot is a common foot complaint, which is caused by a fungal infection. The top layers of affected skin continually peel away, revealing a red, inflamed and very itchy patch of skin. Flare-ups, when painful blisters may appear, can often be linked with warm weather and damp feet, so it is important to keep your feet cool and dry.

Strict foot hygiene is essential. After washing the feet, make sure that they are dried completely. Pay particular attention to the skin between the toes, as the most common site of infection is between the fourth and fifth toes. Wear only socks made from natural fibres and when possible give your feet a break from wearing shoes altogether.

BLISTER BUSTER

Combine infusions of comfrey and witch hazel and dab on to heal blisters.

Foot Baths and Balms

MUSTARD FOOT BATH

This is wonderful bath for cold winter evenings. It warms you up and helps to prevent you from getting colds and flu.

75 g/5 tbsp mustard powder
2 tbsp dried spearmint
600 ml/1 pt/2½ cups water
5 drops eucalyptus citradora

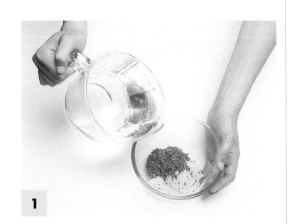

1

1 Make an infusion using the mustard, spearmint and water.

2 Add the eucalyptus oil. Use immediately by adding to a foot bath filled with warm water.

REFRESHING FOOT FIZZ

Create your own foot spa.

2 drops essential oil
100 g/3 tbsp sodium bicarbonate
15 ml/½ fl oz/1 tbsp citric acid

1 For the essential oil, choose between the combinations lemon and lime, geranium and orange, and peppermint and black pepper.

2 Dissolve all the ingredients together in hot water in a large bowl for the feet.

VERRUCAS

Try these local remedies; if they do not help, seek professional advice.

• Garlic macerated oil: dab on daily

• Fresh dandelion sap: squeeze the milky sap found inside the dandelion stalk on to the verruca daily

• Thuja tincture: dab on daily

• Tea tree essential oil: dab on daily

Foot Baths and Balms

MULLED WINTER WARMER

This is a warming and deeply relaxing foot bath which slowly increases circulation to cold feet. Rosehip and hibiscus tea bags can be used as a convenient alternative to the loose herbs.

1 tbsp dried rosehips
2 tbsp dried hibiscus
1 tsp cloves
1 tsp juniper berries
3 bay leaves, crushed
1 tbsp orange peel, fresh or dried
3 drops ginger essential oil

1 Place all the ingredients in a muslin (cheesecloth) bag and gently stir it in a bowl of boiling water.

2 When the liquid has cooled enough for the skin to bear, immerse your feet.

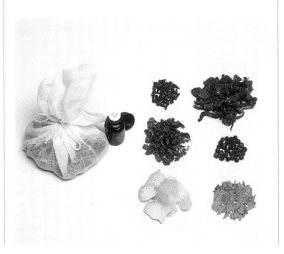

TEA TREE AND THYME FOOT BALM

An antiseptic and healing cream, particularly good for treating athlete's foot. It will last for 6 months if stored in an airtight jar. When you are cleaning the bowl afterwards, heat it to melt excess balm and wipe away with kitchen roll – do not wash it down the drain. These ingredients are sufficient to make 40 g/1½ oz.

10 g/2 tsp beeswax (granules or grated)
45 ml/1½ fl oz/3 tbsp almond oil
15 ml/½ fl oz/1 tbsp wheatgerm oil
5 ml/1 tsp marsh mallow tincture
5 ml/1 tsp comfrey tincture
5 drops thyme essential oil
5 drops tea tree essential oil

1 Heat the beeswax and almond oil in a bowl set over a saucepan of boiling water until the beeswax has melted.

2 Add the wheatgerm oil and the marsh mallow and comfrey tinctures and stir. Remove from the heat and cool slightly.

3 Add the essential oils and mix thoroughly. Pour into a glass jar and allow to set.

FOOT BATH FOR HOT FEET

To 1 tablespoon of Dead Sea Salts add 10 drops of peppermint essential oil. Dissolve in hot water in a bowl for the feet. Also try grapefruit or tea tree essential oils.

Foot Baths and Balms

DOUBLE MINT FOOT CREAM

A cooling and refreshing cream which will gently soften and soothe the skin. These ingredients are sufficient to make 100 g/3½ oz.

10 g/2 tsp cocoa butter
10 g/2 tsp beeswax
30 ml/1 fl oz/2 tbsp almond oil
15 ml/½ fl oz/1 tbsp wheatgerm oil
30 ml/2 tbsp/1 fl oz spearmint infusion
½ tsp borax
10 drops peppermint essential oil

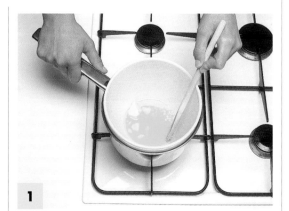

1 Heat the cocoa butter, beeswax and base oils together in a bowl over a saucepan of water until the ingredients have melted.

2 Warm the infusion and dissolve the borax in it.

3 Take the oily mixture off the heat, slowly add the infusion and stir until cool.

4 Add the essential oils and store in a glass jar in the refrigerator. It will keep for at least 2 months.

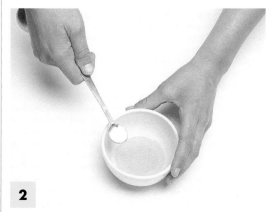

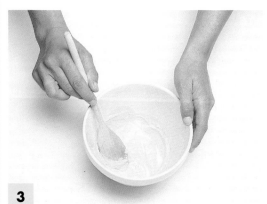

Special Treatments

MYRRH AND MANDARIN FOOT SCRUB

Not only does this scrub effectively remove hard skin, it also softens and protects the delicate skin left behind. The easiest way to crush the pumice stone is to pound it using a pestle and mortar. Both the size of the crushed pumice particles and the overall quantity used depend on how sensitive the soles of your feet are – you may find that with successive batches you are able to tolerate more. These ingredients are sufficient to make 40 g/1½ oz.

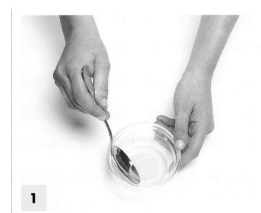

10 g/2 tsp cocoa butter
10 g/2 tsp beeswax (granules or grated)
45 ml/1½ fl oz/3 tbsp apricot kernel oil
30 ml/1 fl oz/2 tbsp marsh mallow infusion
½ tsp borax
1 tbsp crushed pumice stone
12 drops myrrh essential oil
8 drops mandarin essential oil

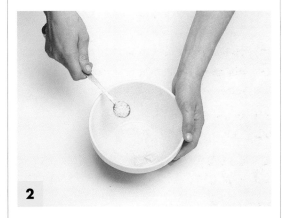

1 Heat the cocoa butter, beeswax and apricot kernel oil together in a bowl set over a saucepan of water until the have melted.

2 Warm the marsh mallow infusion and dissolve the borax in it.

3 Take the oily mixture off the heat. Slowly add the infusion to the oily mixture and stir until cool.

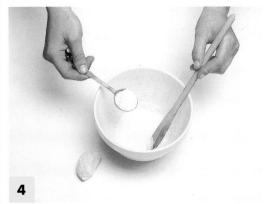

4 Add the pumice stone and the essential oils to the cream and mix thoroughly. It will keep for up to 6 months.

Special Treatments

CHILLI NOT CHILLY

A quick and easy way to warm cold feet is to add cayenne and mustard powder to talcum powder. Both these herbs are rubifacients, which means they stimulate local circulation to the skin and hence add heat. When using before going to bed it is a good idea to wear socks so the powder does not get into the bedding.

LAVENDER AND LEMON FOOT DEODORANT

Witch hazel is an effective astringent, which decreases the flow of secretions from the sweat glands. Lavender kills the bacteria, while lemon acts as a deodorizer. These ingredients are sufficient to make 30 ml/2 tbsp.

30 ml/2 tbsps witch hazel
5 drops lavender essential oil
5 drops lemon essential oil

1 Blend the witch hazel with the essential oils, pour into an atomizer and spray regularly on to clean feet.

2 To ensure an even mix, shake before each application. It will keep for up to 2 months.

BLACKCURRANT AND LEMON FOOT POWDER

This foot powder not only absorbs the secretions but aims to decrease excess sweat production itself, hence treating the source of the odour. After washing and drying your feet thoroughly, sprinkle the powder on and gently rub it in. This powder can also be dusted into footwear for added protection.

1½ g/1 tbsp dried sage
5 g/2 tbsp blackcurrant leaves
10 g/1 tbsp kaolin
5 drops lemon essential oil

1 Grind the sage and blackcurrant into a fine powder, using a pestle and mortar.

2 Add the kaolin and mix thoroughly, then add the lemon essential oil.

3 Store in an old talcum powder dispenser or an empty ground pepper shaker. It will keep for up to 2 months.

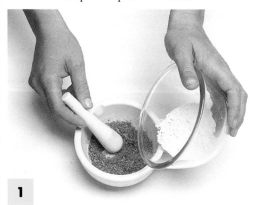

1

Foot Massage

Reflexology is a method of healing that appears to have originated in China. To massage your feet, begin by sitting comfortably, holding one foot. Using mainly your thumbs but also your fingers, apply a good pressure, bit by bit, to the whole surface of the foot. First work your way over the sole of the foot from the toes to the heel. Then work on the top of the foot up to and including the ankle, where other parts of the body are situated. Complete one foot before doing the other. Make sure that your hands remain in contact with the foot throughout the massage.

Any tender spot can be said to represent tension, or possibly illness, in the corresponding organ. Apply a steady pressure for 30 minutes to the painful spot, working around it and coming back to it again and again until any pain has been worked through. If you are performing reflexology on someone else, remember to be gentle and responsive.

FOOT MASSAGE OIL

To make the massage base, combine 90 ml/ 3 fl oz/6 tbsp of almond oil with 10 ml/2 tsp of wheatgerm oil. Add one of the suggested combinations of essential oil listed below:
• Morning blend: 10 drops basil, 5 drops orange, 10 drops sandalwood, 5 drops myrrh
• Evening blend: 5 drops lavender, 10 drops ylang ylang
• Restorative: 5 drops tea tree, 10 drops lavender

REFLEXOLOGY CHART

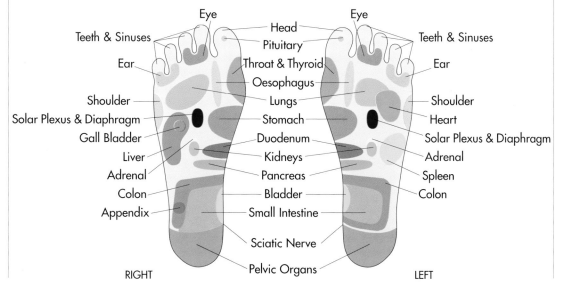

Eye · Head · Eye
Teeth & Sinuses · Pituitary · Teeth & Sinuses
Ear · Throat & Thyroid · Ear
Oesophagus
Shoulder · Lungs · Shoulder
Solar Plexus & Diaphragm · Stomach · Heart
Gall Bladder · Duodenum · Solar Plexus & Diaphragm
Liver · Kidneys · Adrenal
Adrenal · Pancreas · Spleen
Colon · Bladder · Colon
Appendix · Small Intestine
Sciatic Nerve
RIGHT · Pelvic Organs · LEFT

77

Body Care

*Too often we step quickly from under the
shower with barely a thought to the drying
effects of soaps and water on our skin. Use
the recipes that follow to exfoliate and
smooth your skin. Massage your skin with
fragrant lotions to soften and refresh it,
and protect it from the harmful rays of the
sun with some easily prepared oils.*

Most of us don't feel satisfied with what we look like, so it's probably worth remembering that we are more likely to be critical of our own bodies than anybody else is. However, it is worth enjoying looking after ourselves. Exercise not only helps us look good, it makes us feel good, circulating oxygen round the body to re-energize the cells. Pamper yourself, too, by making a special body scrub specifically suited to your skin requirements, or a lotion with carefully chosen essential oils.

Body Brushing

Body brushing will help your body to eliminate toxins by speeding up lymphatic drainage and stimulating the circulation to the skin. Using a cactus fibre body brush or sisal mitt, brush upwards towards the body on your arms and legs, and in towards the centre of your body across the buttocks, small of your back, upper chest and abdomen. Use a firm, sweeping movement without scratching your skin. Do this for five minutes every morning as part of your cleansing routine. If you suffer from cellulite, body brushing and massaging in Neal's Yard Remedies Cellulite Oil daily can really help.

Deodorants

The aluminium compounds that are used in antiperspirants dry up the epidermis and prevent the sweat leaving the body. By combining with the mucus-like substances found in sweat they form a plug which blocks the exit to the sweat duct. Rather than an antiperspirant, it is far better to use a deodorant which inhibits the bacterial growth in the sweat and masks the odour these bacteria produce. The Lemon and Coriander Deodorant on page 82 reduces the number of bacteria which are actually present under the arms. For the armpits, gently rub on ¼ lemon after the juice has been squeezed out – it is the lemon pith that is an effective deodorant.

CELLULITE OIL

With regular use, this oil helps to eliminate toxins from fatty tissues of the body and break down cellulite. Massage in after a warm bath or shower. These ingredients are sufficient to make 100 ml/3½ fl oz. It will keep for up to 12 months.

40 ml/2½ tbsp soya oil
40 ml/2½ tbsp almond oil
20 ml/4 tsp wheatgerm oil
5 drops lemon essential oil
5 drops olibanum essential oil
2 drops juniper essential oil
2 drops black pepper essential oil
5 drops sandalwood essential oil
5 drops sweet orange essential oil
2 drops eucalyptus essential oil

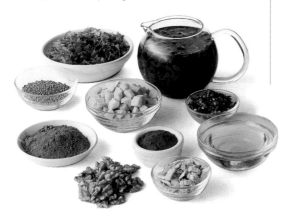

Body Scrubs and Splashes

HONEY AND ORANGE BODY SCRUB

An exfoliating body scrub, especially good for dry skin. These ingredients are sufficient to make 40 g/1½ oz.

10 g/1 tbsp kaolin
30 g/2 tbsp ground rice
5 ml/1 tsp orange flower water or orange blossom infusion
15 ml/1 tbsp clear honey, warmed
1 drop orange essential oil
1 drop geranium essential oil
1 drop juniper essential oil

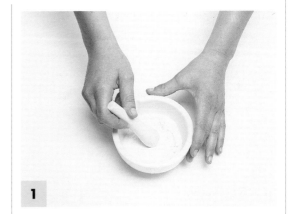

1 Pound the kaolin and ground rice together with a pestle and mortar.

2 Add the orange flower water or infusion and slightly heated honey to the dry mixture and mix thoroughly until fully combined.

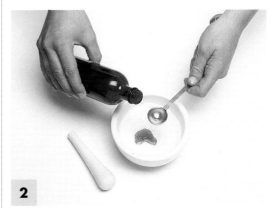

3 Add the essential oils and mix in thoroughly.

4 To use, mix with a small amount of water on the palm of the hand and massage lightly into the skin with small circular movements. Rinse off with warm water. It will keep for up to 2 months.

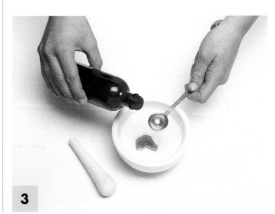

Body Scrubs and Splashes

EXFOLIATING BODY SCRUB

Oats are very cleansing and bran actually penetrates the pores of the skin, removing deeply ingrained dirt and grease. For skin that tends to be oily, use crushed aduki beans and oatmeal. Ground almonds can be added for a more nourishing effect.

20 g/4 tbsp bran
40 g/4 tbsp oats

1 Place the bran and oats in a muslin (cheesecloth) bag and hang it from the tap so that the bath water runs through the bag.

2 When you are in the bath rub your skin with the bag, paying particular attention to areas of dry, hard skin.

BODY SPLASH

This is a delicious body splash/spray that will keep you smelling wonderful! These ingredients are sufficient to make 100 ml/3½ fl oz.

80 ml/5⅓ tbsp distilled water
10 ml/2 tsp aloe vera
5 ml/1 tsp orange flower water
2 drops patchouli essential oil
1 drop geranium essential oil

1 Combine the ingredients and store in a 100 ml/3½ fl oz bottle. It will keep for up to 2 months.

2 Apply with an atomizer, shaking before use.

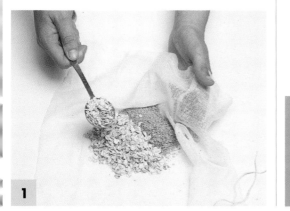

1

EXFOLIATION
Exfoliation stimulates lymphatic drainage and promotes circulation. It also encourages skin cell production and improves the condition of the skin.

Moisturizing Skin Oils

The following recipes all make 100 ml/3½ fl oz/scant ½ cup.
All you need do is blend the essential oils with the base oils.
Store in dark glass bottles away from sunlight. They will keep
for up to 30 months.

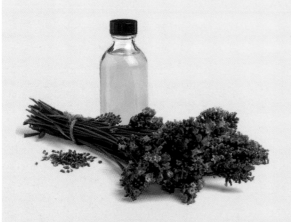

STIMULATING SKIN CONDITIONING OIL

An energizing massage oil.

20 ml/4 tsp almond oil
20 ml/4 tsp sunflower oil
20 ml/4 tsp coconut oil
20 ml/4 tsp grapeseed oil
10 ml/2 tsp avocado oil
10 ml/2 tsp wheatgerm oil
10 drops lavender essential oil
10 drops peppermint essential oil
10 drops juniper essential oil
10 drops rosemary essential oil

SOOTHING SKIN CONDITIONING OIL

A relaxing, calming massage oil.

20 ml/4 tsp almond oil
20 ml/4 tsp sunflower oil
20 ml/4 tsp coconut oil
20 ml/4 tsp grapeseed oil
10 ml/2 tsp avocado oil
10 ml/2 tsp wheatgerm oil
10 drops geranium essential oil
10 drops bergamot essential oil
10 drops lavender essential oil
10 drops cypress essential oil

GERANIUM AND ORANGE MASSAGE OIL

*A light, fragrant massage oil, suitable
for all skin types.*

40 ml/2½ tbsp soya oil
40 ml/2½ tbsp almond oil
20 ml/4 tsp wheatgerm oil
20 drops geranium essential oil
20 drops orange essential oil

Special Treatments

To make these treatment oils simply blend the essential oils into the base oils. Both recipes make 100 ml/3½ fl oz. To protect the essential oils from sunlight store them in dark glass bottles. They will keep for up to 12 months.

ANTI-PARASITIC OIL

This oil contains parasiticide essential oils and can be used to prevent and/or get rid of parasites living on the skin, such as scabies.

100 ml/3½ fl oz/scant ½ cup almond oil
10 drops palmarosa essential oil
10 drops lavendin or lavender essential oil
10 drops wild thyme essential oil
10 drops rosemary
  essential oil
10 drops lemon
  essential oil

GINGER AND JUNIPER WARMING OIL

This is a deeply warming rubbing oil, perfect for aching muscles and areas of the body affected by the cold. It will also ease the pain of rheumatism. Massage it in deeply to affected parts and keep the area warm.

80 ml/5⅓ tbsp almond oil
20 ml/2 tsp wheatgerm oil
5 drops ginger essential oil
5 drops juniper essential oil
5 drops lavender essential oil
5 drops rosemary essential oil
5 drops sage essential oil

Special Treatments

SPRAY-ON INSECT REPELLENT

These ingredients are sufficient to make 25 ml/1 fl oz.

25 ml/5 tsp lavender flower water
1 drop sandalwood essential oil
2 drops citronella essential oil
3 drops eucalyptus citriadora essential oil

1 Add the essential oils to the lavender flower water and store in a glass bottle.

2 Shake before use and spray on the skin using an atomizer. It will keep for 6 months.

INSECT REPELLENT – ESSENTIAL OIL BLEND

Where the skin is hot or sensitive, replace half the lavender flower water with aloe vera.

1 drop cinnamon essential oil
1 drop lemon grass essential oil
2 drops orange essential oil
2 drops wild thyme essential oil
4 drops lavender essential oil
4 drops pine essential oil
4 drops eucalyptus citriadora essential oil
5 drops citronella essential oil
100 ml/3½ fl oz/scant ½ cup
lavender flower water

1 Mix the essential oils with the flower water.

2 Shake well before use and apply with an atomizer spray. It will keep for 6 months.

LEMON AND CORIANDER DEODORANT

A refreshing and effective deodorant. These ingredients are sufficient to make 100 ml/3½ fl oz.

90 ml/6 tbsp witch hazel
10 ml/2 tsp vegetable glyderine
2 drops clove essential oil
2 drops coriander essential oil
5 drops grapefruit essential oil
2 drops lavender essential oil
10 drops lemon essential oil
5 drops lime essential oil
5 drops palmarosa essential oil

1 Mix the witch hazel and vegetable glycerine together.

2 Add the essential oils and mix in.

3 Store in a dark glass bottle, preferably with an atomizer spray, for up to 6 months.

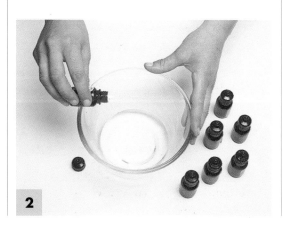

2

Body Powders

CALENDULA POWDER

Body powders help the skin to remain dry and prevent chafing. This is for delicate and sensitive skin.

20 g/2 tbsp kaolin
5 drops calendula tincture
5 drops lemon essential oil

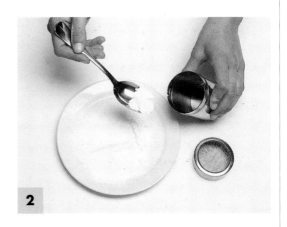

1 Sift the kaolin evenly on to a plate.

2 Mix the tincture and essential oil and spray on to the kaolin, using an atomizer pump.

3 Store in an old talc dispenser or empty ground pepper shaker. It will keep for up to 6 months.

GERANIUM AND ORANGE POWDER

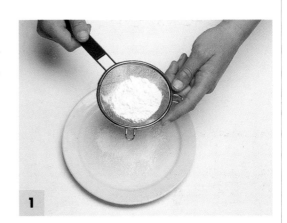

5 drops geranium essential oil
5 drops orange essential oil
20 g/¾ oz/3 tbsp cornflour (cornstarch)

1 Sift the cornstarch evenly on to a plate.

2 Mix the oils and spray on to the cornflour (cornstarch), using an atomizer pump.

3 Store in an old talc dispenser or empty ground pepper shaker. It will keep for up to 6 months.

Sun Products

These two sun oils are nourishing and conditioning to the skin – but remember that the sun is damaging, even when oil is applied. Simply blend all the oils together and store them in dark glass bottles.

SESAME SUN OIL

Sesame oil does offer a low degree of protection against the sun's rays, and this oil will nourish dry skin. The ingredients will make 100 ml/3½ fl oz. It will keep for up to 12 months.

40 ml/2½ tbsp sesame oil
40 ml/2½ tbsp coconut oil
20 ml/4 tsp grapeseed oil
40 drops petitgrain essential oil
5 drops lavender essential oil

LIME AND COCONUT SUN OIL

This oil offers no protection and is only suitable for dark skin which tans very easily, or for use after exposure to the sun. These ingredients will make 60 ml/4 tbsp. It will keep for up to 12 months.

10 ml/2 tsp wheatgerm oil
20 g/¾ oz cocoa butter
50 ml/3⅓ tbsp coconut oil
5 drops benzoin tincture
10 drops lime essential oil

Chamomile blue is an excellent anti-inflammatory oil, which is good to use on sensitive skin.

OILS FOR SUNBURNT SKIN

The following recipes can be used to heal and condition sunburnt skin – but remember that you should try to avoid overexposure to the sun in the first place.

CALENDULA AND ST JOHN'S WORT SOOTHING OIL

Calendula heals and soothes the skin, while St John's wort acts by calming stimulated nerve tissue, and is often used in after-sun skin-care products.

5 ml/1 tsp calendula oil
5 ml/1 tsp St John's wort oil
2 drops lavender essential oil

1 Mix the ingredients together and store in a dark glass bottle for up to 6 months.

ALOE VERA COOLER

This is an excellent lotion for taking the heat out of sunburnt and damaged skin. Aloe vera soothes and softens the skin. Calendula is added for its healing and soothing properties.

10 ml/2 tsp liquid aloe vera
15 drops calendula tincture

1 Mix the ingredients together and store in a dark glass bottle for up to 6 months.

Sun Products

SOOTHING OINTMENT FOR SUNBURNT SKIN

Another way of applying treatment to sunburnt skin is to add the essential oils and tinctures to an ointment base ,which is slowly absorbed into the skin. It will keep for up to 30 months.

1 drop chamomile blue essential oil
4 drops lavender essential oil
15 drops calendula tincture
25 g/1 oz ointment base

1 Combine the oils and tincture and add to the ointment base.

COCOA BUTTER BODY LOTION

A soothing and moisturizing body lotion suitable for skin which has been exposed to the sun and also to use as a general skin conditioner. This recipe makes a 100ml/3½ fl oz bottle.

15 g/½ oz cocoa butter
1 tsp lanolin
75 ml/5 tbsp wheatgerm oil
5 ml/1 tsp clear honey
45 ml/3 tbsp water
½ tsp borax
5 drops benzoin tincture
5 drops sandalwood essential oil
5 drops helichrysum essential oil
5 drops ylang ylang essential oil

1 Melt the cocoa butter, lanolin and wheat germ oil in a bowl set over a pan of water.

2 Heat the water and dissolve the honey and borax in it.

3 Add the water mixture to the oil mixture one tablespoon at a time, whisking.

4 Add the essential oils and benzoin tincture.

5 Store in a glass bottle in the refrigerator for up to 3 weeks. Shake before use.

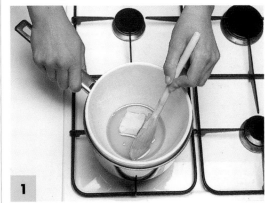

1

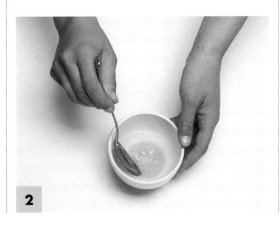

2

Bath Bombs

Opinion is divided as to whether an invigorating shower or a bath is best, but if you have a shower as well as a bathtub the ideal is to sluice off all those dead cells, bacteria and the pollutants before you luxuriate in a hot bath – which of course you can always share if you're concerned about using so much water! Choose a blend of essential oils to fragrance the bath, or add in one of the following recipes. Fill the bath and take time to relax – try candlelight for a really soothing environment.

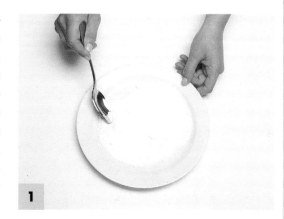

BATH BOMBS

This hedonistic recipe will turn your bath into a fragrant jacuzzi. These ingredients will make one or two bombs. They will keep for up to 2 months in a sealed container.

80 g/3 tbsp sodium bicarbonate
15 ml/1 tbsp citric acid
10 drops essential oil of your choice
(see page 89)

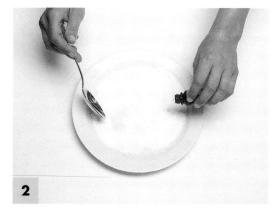

1 Mix the sodium bicarbonate and citric acid together on a plate.

2 Sprinkle the sodium bicarbonate mixture with essential oil.

3 This powder can be sprinkled into the bath or moulded by compression into a solid block. We used camera film cases as a mould. Add the powder or block just before you step into the bath.

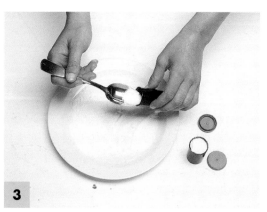

Milk Baths

Milk supplies us with a high content of vitamins, minerals and calcium. It is easily absorbed by the skin and is just as effective used externally. Bathing in milk leaves the skin feeling conditioned and moisturized, but as the smell of milk in the bath can be unpleasant it is best combined with essential oils.

CLEOPATRA'S BEAUTY BATH

These ingredients are sufficient for one bath.

**100 ml/3½ fl oz/scant ½ cup full-fat milk
(cow's, sheep's or goat's)
5 ml/1 tsp clear honey
5 drops jasmine absolute
5 drops ylang ylang essential oil**

1 Heat the milk gently in a saucepan and add the honey.

2 Take off the heat and add the essential oils.

3 Use immediately by adding to a ready-run warm bath.

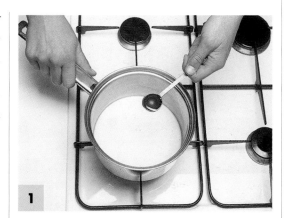

1

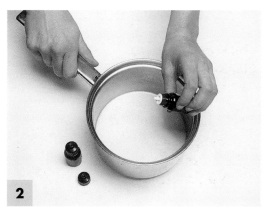

2

TROPICAL MILK BATH

For one nourishing and relaxing bath, pour 45 g/3 tbsp powdered coconut milk into a ready-run warm bath, lie back and think of palm trees. A good variation on this is to leave a vanilla pod and a tonka bean in the coconut powder to create a tropical fragrance.

ESSENTIAL OILS FOR BATHS

Relaxing: 5 drops lavender essential oil and 5 drops ylang ylang essential oil

Refreshing: 5 drops bergamot essential oil and 5 drops grapefruit essential oil

Milk Baths

KIDS' MILKSHAKE BATH

This is a great recipe for children with sensitive skin. These ingredients are sufficient for one bath.

100 ml/3½ fl oz/scant ½ cup full-fat milk
(cow's, sheep's or goat's)
5 ml/1 tsp natural food colouring

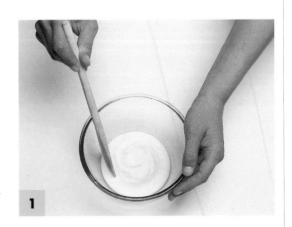

1. Mix the milk with the food colouring in a bowl and then pour into a warm bath.

ESSENTIAL OIL BATHS

Adding essential oils to the bath is a wonderfully pleasurable and very popular way of using them. The warmth of the water encourages relaxation and also enables the essential oils to penetrate the skin. The oils should only be added to the water once the bath has been run, as the heat will encourage their evaporation.

Only the essential oils that are non-irritant, such as Roman chamomile and lavender, should be added directly to the bath; just add 4–6 drops of essential oil and swirl the water around before stepping in. All other essential oils should be diluted first in a carrier because they will not fully disperse in the water and their molecules may well come into direct contact with the skin and mucous membranes. Suitable carriers include base oils, specially prepared bath oil bases, which have a dispersant added, and full-fat milk.

To prepare a bath using a carrier, mix 4–6 drops of essential oil to an eggcupful of milk or 10 ml/2 tsp of oil, add the mixture to the bath and swirl the water before stepping in. Good base oils to use are soya, almond and grapeseed.

For a rather more nourishing effect, add a teaspoon of evening primrose oil or jojoba oil. Oil blends can also be mixed with Dead Sea Salts or sea salt before adding to the bath.

* Stimulating: Bergamot, coriander, cypress, grapefruit, juniper, lemon, lime, peppermint, pine, rosemary.

* Uplifting: Bergamot, clary sage, geranium, jasmine, mandarin, melissa, neroli, olibanum, orange, palmarosa, rose.

* Relaxing: Chamomile, clary sage, geranium, lavender, marjoram, neroli, rose, sandal wood, vetiver, ylang ylang.

* Deep cleansing: Cypress, grapefruit, juniper, lemon, tea tree.

Herbal Infusions

SEAWEED AND ARNICA BATH INFUSION

This combines an infusion of mineral-rich seaweed with arnica tincture and essential oils of lemon, pine and juniper to create a refreshing and revitalizing bath.

½ tsp bladderwrack
1 tsp comfrey leaf
2 tsp juniper berries
500 ml/18 fl oz/2¼ cups water
2 heaped tsp sea salt
5 drops arnica tincture
2 drops pine essential oil
2 drops lavender essential oil
2 drops lemon essential oil
2 drops juniper essential oil

1 Make an infusion from the bladderwrack, comfrey, juniper berries and water.

2 Add salt and stir, then add the arnica tincture and essential oils.

3 Use immediately by adding to a ready-run warm bath.

ANTI-CELLULITE BATH INFUSION

With a combination of a careful diet, massage, exercise and dry brushing it is possible to banish cellulite. Adding this diuretic and stimulating infusion to the bath will also help.

½ tsp bladderwrack
2 tsp fennel seeds
1 tsp celery seeds
500 ml/18 fl oz/2¼ cups water
2 tsp sea salt
2 drops fennel essential oil
2 drops juniper essential oil
2 drops eucalyptus
2 drops black pepper

1 Make an infusion from the bladderwrack, fennel and celery seeds and the water.

2 Mix in the salt and add the essential oils.

3 Use immediately by adding it to a ready-run warm bath.

When a recipe calls for water,
use filtered, bottled or distilled water
or water that has been boiled and allowed to cool.

Herbal Infusions

ROSE AND ROSEHIP INFUSION

*This infusion makes a good skin tonic
for dry and sensitive skin.*

**500 ml/18 fl oz/2¼ cups water
2 tsp dried rose petals/buds
1 tsp dried rosehips
1 tsp salt
5 ml/1 tsp cider vinegar
5 drops calendula tincture
8 drops rose essential oil
2 drops geranium essential oil**

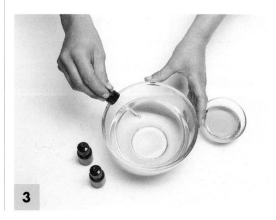

1 Make an infusion using the rosehips, rose petals and water. Strain.

2 Add the rest of the ingredients.

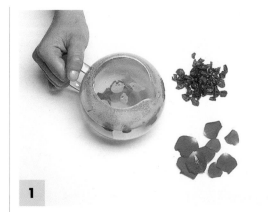

3 Use immediately by adding to a warm bath.

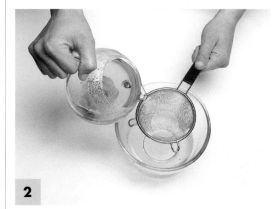

Herbal Infusions

ALOE VERA AND LAVENDER INFUSION

This is cooling and soothing, perfect for sensitive skin which has been exposed to the sun.

2 tsp lavender flowers
2 tsp chamomile flowers
500 ml/18 fl oz/2¼ cups water
30 ml/2 tbsp aloe vera juice
10 drops lavender essential oil

1 Make an infusion of the lavender, chamomile and water.

2 Add the aloe vera and lavender essential oil.

3 Use immediately by adding to a ready-run warm bath.

LEMON GRASS AND BAY LEAF INFUSION

This infusion is suitable after a bout of sporting activity or any over-exertion.

2 tsp bay leaves
1 tsp rosemary
500 ml/18 fl oz/2¼ cups water
5 drops lemon grass essential oil

1 Make an infusion of the bay leaves and rosemary and the water.

2 Add the lemon grass essential oil.

3 Use immediately by adding to a ready-run warm bath.

SITZ BATHS

A sitz bath is an excellent way of treating haemorrhoids, thrush, pruritis, stitches following childbirth and so on. Half-fill a large bowl or small bath with warm water. Use the same method of dilution as for baths and sit in the water for 10 minutes. Adding tea tree oil to a sitz bath is the classic treatment for thrush.

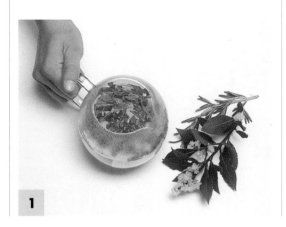

1

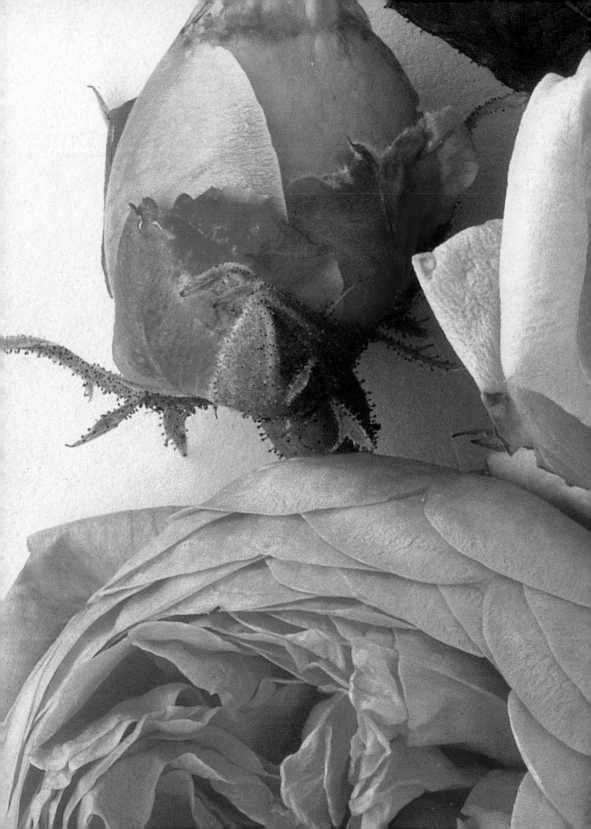

Perfumery and Fragrancing

Commercial perfume producers may choose from

3,000 individual elements to create a single

perfume, but such complexity is not necessary.

Using just a few essential oils and learning how to

combine the individual fragrances into a subtle,

balanced whole is not difficult. Simply refer to the

guidelines on the pages that follow.

We are so accustomed to interpreting the world we live in by what we see and hear that it is easy to underestimate the part played by our sense of smell. We would be surprised to realize how greatly the way we feel about the people we meet and the places we visit is affected by our sense of smell. Our memory stores up associations of fragrances, and the art of fragrancing is to evoke these connections.

As we breathe in air through our noses, fragrant molecules are drawn up past the smell receptor cells, which react to each new odour. This reaction triggers an electrical signal to the part of the brain that is associated with feelings and emotions, so it is not surprising that what we smell connects us to the feelings we associate with it. Research has shown that the aromas of certain essential oils will bring about specific mood changes. We are beginning to see the potential in essential oils for effecting how we feel – the floral oils, for example, have been shown to be mood enhancing.

We rely more on our olfactory sense than we may first think. As babies, we learn to recognize our mother by her smell. Imagine a warm sunny walk through a meadow and not being able to smell the fresh, green fragrance. Try walking into a coffee shop without the aroma of coffee brewing and freshly cooked pastries! If we were unable to smell, our days would seem drab and dull, and we would feel strangely lost without this sense of connection to our past.

We know that the human ability to distinguish smells is far inferior to that of other animals. For example, the male Emperor moth can detect a female moth over 10 kilometres (6 miles) away; an Alsatian dog has 220 million sense cells in its nose compared to a human with a mere 10 million!

It is interesting that we are largely unaware of our sense of smell and the part that it plays in our lives. We have hardly developed a language to describe what we smell. When it comes to our other senses we have a whole vocabulary to describe what things look like or how they sound, and it is possible that as humans have evolved, the olfactory sense has become less significant. It is known that humans are sexually attracted to each other through the pheromones or body smells that we all possess, but throughout history we have striven to mask these smells and replace them with expensive perfumes, many of which now contain synthetic sexual attractants.

ESSENTIAL OILS

The use of oils goes back a long way in history. Simple equipment used for making essential oils that has been dated as far back as 3000BC has been found in the Indian subcontinent. Oils such as jatamansi and cedarwood were used to excite the senses; eucalyptus was used for its therapeutic properties; olibanum, myrrh and cinnamon were used to raise the level of the soul of the individual and to exalt the spirit. Fragrant oils, waxes and unguents have long been used to enhance the body and add allure. It is said that Cleopatra painted her ship's sails with fragrant oils to attract Mark Antony as he sailed towards her across the Mediterranean. Different religious traditions around the world still burn oils and incense in places of worship.

Towards the end of ancient times, condiments and spices began to be used more and more widely, and trade in these commodities developed around the world. Oils such as ylang ylang, vetiver and patchouli came to be produced, marking the first stages in perfumery as we know it.

The fragrance of a plant is present in minute glands. If you pick a leaf of peppermint and rub it gently between your finger and thumb the familiar mint smell is released when the cell walls containing volatile oils are broken down. Volatile oils are present in plants for different purposes: for example, eucalyptus has insecticidal properties to protect the plants from being eaten by insects or larger animals, while roses contain fragrant oils to attract insects so that pollination can occur, and the frankincense tree produces resin to heal wounds or damage to the tree itself.

Mentha x *piperita*
(peppermint)

The volatile oils are found in different parts of the plant – in the flowers of mimosa, rose and ylang ylang; in the flowers and leaves of peppermint, lavender, rosemary and violet; in the leaves and stems of geranium, thyme and petigrain; in the bark of cinnamon; in the roots of vetiver and ginger; in the fruits of lemon, lime and bergamot; in the resins of frankincense, myrrh and benzoin; in the seeds of dill, fennel and aniseed; and in the wood of cedar, pine and sandalwood.

Most oils are produced by steam distillation. Water is heated and the rising steam passes into a receptacle containing the plant material. The heat causes the fragile oil sacs to break, and the volatile oil passes into the steam. When the steam cools, reverting to a liquid, the water and oil separate and the oil is drawn off. The water can be used as a flower water or 'hydrolat'. Steam distillation is a very similar process, but the water does not actually touch the plant. This is preferable because the plant is less likely to be damaged.

In the case of citrus fruit, the volatile oil is found in the peel and is extracted by expression after the peel has been removed from the fruit. New types of extraction processes involving carbon dioxide and nitrogen are now being used, and these cause even less damage to the plant and are less energy consuming. They may be among the extraction processes of the future.

As the art of distilling oils developed, so did the art of fragrancing as we now know it.

Grasse, in the south of France, became recognized as the centre of a perfume industry, and oils were produced from locally grown crops such as jasmine, lavender and narcissus. Today, crops are grown and distilled all over the world.

Oils of any one type can vary enormously depending on the variety of the plant, the climate in which it is grown and the way the oil is extracted. The yields can range from plant to plant. Lavender produces around 1 kg (2.2 lb) of oil to 100 kg (220 lb) of flowers and leaves, whereas violets may produce 3 g (less than ⅛ oz) of oil to 100 kg (220 lb) of flowers!

Oils are produced for different purposes, and different qualities are required for the various industries that use them. In the flavouring industry, for example, oils are added to confectionery and other foods. One of the largest crop of oils is peppermint – for example, in 1996 over 5.5 thousand tonnes of the species *Mentha arvensis* and *Mentha* x *piperita* were produced in the USA alone. Incidentally, peppermint oil is also widely used in the pharmaceutical industry.

The perfume industry is the other main user of essential oils, although they are not the only fragrance ingredients used.

THE INGREDIENTS YOU USE

Whatever you are making, the ingredients you use will give your product its basic look and fragrance. This is why it is always worth making certain you use good quality ingredients. If, for example, you use cheap malt vinegar in a hair rinse, it is likely to smell like something from a chip shop! Similarly, using over-ripe fruit in a face mask will make the mask less effective, and it will smell less fresh.

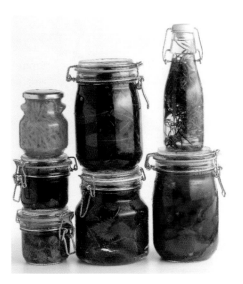

It is worthwhile experimenting with your products by varying the ingredients and thus changing the colour, texture and fragrance. Make sure that you have thought through the reason for including each ingredient. It is best to be guided by the properties of the plant, which may appear to be a simple approach, but it seems to be the best policy, and it is certainly what we try to adhere to at Neal's Yard Remedies. In this way, the formulation has a clear function and the fragrance always seems to be appropriate. If it doesn't seem right, it could quite easily be because one or other of the ingredients is not the best to use.

BASE OILS

The fragrance of the base oils will vary. Wheatgerm oil has a strong, earthy smell;

hazelnut oil gives off a delicious, nutty odour, which can significantly enhance the depth of a fragrance; olive and sesame oils are also distinctive; and oils such as grapeseed, almond and sunflower are lighter. When you are creating your own mixtures, it is probably best, in the first instance, to be guided by the purpose of your creation. Thus, if you want an enriching face cream with a high nutritive base, use oils such as avocado and almond, which will create a base cream that smells rather buttery.

MACERATED OILS

Generally, these oils have quite a mild fragrance of the particular herb used – unless you are macerating something like garlic! They can be added to a mixture and, in the case of St John's wort or carrot macerates, are more likely to alter the colour than the fragrance.

TINCTURES

The main aroma of tinctures is generally that of alcohol, which will evaporate away, leaving behind the herbal odour. This is not generally very strong and will not tend to dominate a mixture, although tinctures will colour the product.

INFUSIONS

An infusion is a water extract of plants, which is similar to a tincture but which will add a mild, herby fragrance to your mixture. Depending on the strength of the infusion and the colour of the plant, the look of the resulting cream or shampoo will vary significantly, much less than the smell, unless you use something like seaweed, which is a wonderful ingredient, rich in minerals, but nevertheless strong smelling!

FINDING THE APPROPRIATE FRAGRANCE

It is worth remembering that we do, in general, have an idea of how things should smell. The science behind fragrancing is to recognize what we expect different products to smell like, and to design a fragrance that is appropriate. Often a fragrance is used to mask unpleasant odours, but this will rarely be the case when you are making simple recipes for your skin and hair, which will, if no essential oils are added, smell of the ingredients, rather than oily or buttery.

Getting to know essential oils by actually using them is the best way to gain the basic memory building blocks. Start by learning about their properties and what contribution they can make to the function of your products.

When you make a product to stimulate and nourish the hair, you would probably expect it to smell rather 'herby'. Rosemary is an excellent essential oil to use for a hair product, but if you had decided to use, say, orange, you might not believe that it was quite

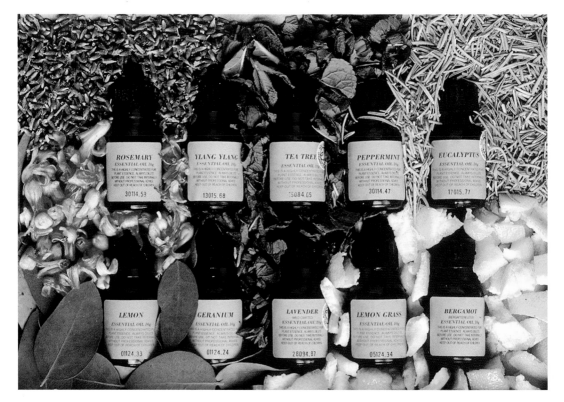

as effective, simply from the fragrance, and in this instance, your instinct would be quite correct. Orange, however, blends very well with other oils, notably spicy or sweet oils, to lighten or lift fragrance. Be guided by its function as a good toning and detoxifying essential oil, which will help you to recognize when to include it. Similarly, when you smell tea tree or eucalyptus in a product, you automatically associate it with an antiseptic function.

THE CLASSIFICATION OF OILS

Unlike other senses, the sense of smell does not have many descriptive words connected with it – smells are never big, red or loud!

Adjectives like these belong to the vocabulary of the other senses. We tend to describe smells by referring to a past memory or by connecting a smell to something that we feel is similar.

Perfumers have created a language specifically to describe fragrances. They use an analogy with musical notation, referring to levels and types of fragrance as notes. Top notes are seen as being sharp (in Chinese terms 'yin') – for example, bergamot and lemon. In a blend, the smell of these oils will be the first to be perceived and the first to disappear, leaving the next level, or middle notes. This group has a more even, balanced odour. It is the heart of a fragrance, or its deep note, and gives the body of fragrant blend – as with geranium, cinnamon and marjoram, for example. Oils described as having a base note, such as vanilla, vetiver or patchouli, can be used as fixatives. They hold a fragrance together, giving it depth and endurance.

CREATING A PERFUME

Creating a balanced perfume requires a blend from each group of oils. A single perfume may be made up of as many as fifty ingredients, which have been selected from the 3,000 that are available, not all of which are natural. Since it was discovered how to create different fragrances using synthetics and extracts from other oils, it is increasingly common to find perfumes with only a small percentage of natural essential oil. In some instances this is a positive development, because in the past, animal extracts were used. Animals such as the civet cat, the musk deer and the beaver suffered in the pursuit of the very expensive ingredients the animals produced.

Perfumes are classified into odour groups. Perfumers will use terms like citrus, woody, green, floral, spicy, amber and leathery to describe a raw material. It is useful to have a basic awareness of these different fragrance classifications so that you can create a balanced fragrance. More important, however, is always to use good quality, reliable ingredients. As you spend more time working with essential oils, you will acquire a memory of them, and then making a fragrance will simply become a work of the imagination – visualization.

It is worth reiterating that being clear about what you want to achieve is most important. At Neal's Yard Remedies we ask ourselves what we would like to achieve from a product before asking how we would like it to be. This isn't the only way, but it is important to clarify what the product is for and how you would like it to smell. Once this is established, make a preliminary selection of oils. Again, when it comes to developing our own ideas, choices will be made according to the function we envisage for the finished product. For example, one project was to create a foaming bath, which we wanted to be as effective as possible. It was intended to soothe aching muscles, to help with tiredness and to leave the user feeling rejuvenated. Choosing the ingredients was not that difficult – pine, lemon and juniper essential oils, arnica tincture and infusions of seaweed, juniper berries and comfrey. Balancing the fragrance of the product was more difficult, however, and we would proceed in a similar way to that outlined below.

Once the purpose of the product has been established, prepare some smelling strips. These can be made by cutting blotting paper into thin strips. It will be useful to number the strips. Arrange the oils around you for easy reference and place a drop of each oil you think you would like to include on a smelling strip. This will give you a very broad idea of how well the oils work together. The next step is to record the combination of oils used. Make a note of the number of the strip you have used and then write down what you have just done.

If you like your newly created fragrance, try mixing it in a small beaker and adjust the quantities until it seems more balanced and no particular oil overpowers another. Creating a blend by using a top note oil, a middle note and a base note will give you a fragrance in which each individual oil is enhanced by the others. Each oil remains distinct yet is a part of the whole. Often a mix that seems so promising when you begin becomes confused and messy, so don't be afraid to start again!

To help you choose the oils to add to the product you are making you need to consider two main factors – what purpose the oil will have and what mood do you want to create? The answers to these two questions are not necessarily different, but it is worth defining your expectations at the outset so that you make the correct choices.

DILUTIONS

Following are rough guides to the proportions in which the fragrance you have just made should be added into the mixture. If you wish to keep your mixture as a perfume, the base can be either alcohol or jojoba.

ALCOHOL

As with making tinctures (see page 21), it is probably best to use vodka or purchase alcohol from the chemist. This is especially appropriate when creating a perfume. The blend of essential oils should be added so that it forms between 3 and 8 per cent of the whole.

FLOWER WATERS

These products already contain essential oils, but will allow an extra one per cent of oil blend to be added. These are excellent for room sprays, insect repellents and so on when a predominant water base is required.

A blended fragrance of essential oils will be therapeutically effective above 2 per cent. It is best to keep below this level unless a specific effect is required. Don't forget that oils are readily absorbed through the skin.

CREAM BASE

Making your own cream is described on page 24. The base will smell of the ingredients, so you will need to consider this when you come to add a fragrance. A creamy, honey base will be enhanced by a sweet, floral blend of oils, and this would be appropriate for a rich night cream. A soothing aftersun cream with aloe vera and chamomile in the base may well benefit from something lighter and a more cooling fragrance. Add your fragrance at a percentage of 1–3 of the total.

Use the following charts to help you select essential oils to blend together to make your own fragrance. Select an oil from each of the three groups – to provide top, middle and base notes – using the suggestions in the second column to create a well-balanced mixture that you can use in other recipes.

The charts on the following pages 103-5 give guidance and suggestions for making your own fragrances to suit your mood in general, but can also be used for self-help aromatherapy. Check the far-right column for the overall therapeutic effect you wish to achieve.

ESSENTIAL OIL	BLENDS WELL WITH	THERAPEUTIC USE	EFFECT
TOP NOTES			
BASIL	Bergamot, chamomile, clary sage, geranium, lavender, lemongrass, marjoram, rose	Nerve tonic, balancing, reviving, strengthening	Relaxing, uplifting
BERGAMOT	Lavender, melissa, rosemary	Nerve tonic	Uplifting
CARDAMON	Bergamot, cedarwood, clove, frankincense, orange, sandalwood, ylang ylang	Digestive tonic, anti-spasmodic, carminative	Tonifying, calming
CLARY SAGE	Cardamon, coriander, geranium, jasmine, lavender, lemon, rose, sandalwood	Strengthens nervous system, stress, anxiety	Soothing, sedating
CORIANDER	Bergamot, clary sage, frankincense, jasmine, sandalwood	Digestive, mildly warming, tonifying	Aphrodisiac
EUCALYPTUS	Cedarwood, cypress, lavender, lemon, marjoram, pine, tea tree, thyme	Antiseptic, decongestant	Warming, refreshing
GRAPEFRUIT	Citrus oils, clove, cypress, ginger, lavender, neroli, palmarosa, rosemary	Detoxifying, astringent	Refreshing, uplifting
JUNIPER	Citrus oils, cedarwood, cypress, ginger, lavender, pine, rosemary	Stimulates elimination of toxic fluids	Cleansing
LAVENDER	Geranium, rosemary	Stress, jet lag, insomnia	Relaxing, balancing
LEMON	Any	Antiseptic, astringent	Stimulating
MANDARIN	Citrus oils, spicy oils, clary sage, geranium, lavender, neroli	Digestive, peristalsis	Refreshing, uplifting
NEROLI	Citrus oils, clary sage, jasmine, lavender, rosemary	Anxiety, depression, insomnia	Relaxing, calming, uplifting

ESSENTIAL OIL	BLENDS WELL WITH	THERAPEUTIC USE	EFFECT
ORANGE	Citrus oils, spice oils, clary sage, geranium, lavender, myrrh, neroli, rosemary	Sluggish digestion, liver detoxifier	Relaxing, uplifting
PEPPERMINT	Fennel, orange	Digestive, antiseptic	Warming, stimulating
PETIGRAIN	Citrus oils, clary sage, jasmine, lavender, rosemary	Nerve tonic	Uplifting, anti-depressant
PINE	Cedarwood, eucalyptus, juniper, lavender, lemon, marjoram, tea tree	Decongestant, urinary infection, rheumatism	Refreshing, reviving
TEA TREE	Clove, eucalyptus, lavender, lemon, pine, rosemary, thyme	Anti-viral, anti-fungal, antiseptic	Stimulating, tonifying
THYME	Clove, eucalyptus, lavender, lemon, pine	Strongly anti-microbial, strengthens immune system	Warming, stimulating
ESSENTIAL OIL	BLENDS WELL WITH	THERAPEUTIC USE	EFFECT
MIDDLE NOTES			
CEDARWOOD	Bergamot, cypress, frankincense, jasmine, juniper, myrrh, neroli, rosemary, sandalwood, vetiver	Warming, regenerating, tonifying, soothing	Balancing
CINNAMON	Clove, eucalyptus, frankincense, lemon, mandarin, orange	Warming, stimulating, stimulating	Restorative
CLOVE	Bergamot, eucalyptus, lavender, thyme	Warming, stimulating, antiseptic	Stimulating, pain-relieving
GERANIUM	Bergamot, lavender, lemon, marjoram, neroli, orange, palmarosa, rose, sandalwood	Calming, cooling	Calming, uplifting
JASMINE	Bergamot, clary sage, orange, rose, sandalwood, ylang ylang	Increases self-confidence, anti-depressant	Uplifting, relaxing, aphrodisiac

ESSENTIAL OIL	BLENDS WELL WITH	THERAPEUTIC USE	EFFECT
MARJORAM	Bergamot, cypress, eucalyptus, geranium, lavender, orange, rosemary	Relieves aching muscles, period pain	Warming, relaxing
OLIBANUM	Citrus oils, spice oils, basil, cedarwood, myrrh, neroli, pine, sandalwood, vetiver	Tonifying, astringent, anti-inflammatory	Aids meditation
PALMAROSA	Bergamot, cedarwood, geranium, mandarin, rose, sandalwood, ylang ylang	Healing, regenerative	Calming, uplifting, digestive tonic
ROMAN CHAMOMILE	Clary sage, lavender, lemon, rose	Anti-inflammatory	Sedative
ROSE	Bergamot, chamomile, clary sage, geranium, jasmine, lavender, patchouli	Cooling, relaxing, tonifying	Anti-depressant, aphrodisiac
YLANG YLANG	Bergamot, cedarwood, clary sage, jasmine, lemon, rose, sandalwood, vetiver	Treats anxiety, depression, stress, tension	Sedating, calming
BASE NOTES			
BENZOIN	Coriander, cypress, frankincense, jasmine, juniper, lemon, myrrh, rose, sandalwood, spice oils	Skin irritation, poor circulation	Anti-inflammatory, carminative, astringent
PATCHOULI	Cedarwood, geranium, neroli	Anti-depressant, antibacterial, anti-viral	Stimulating, astringent
SANDALWOOD	Bergamot, cedarwood, jasmine, palmarosa, vetiver, ylang ylang	Calming, soothing	Relaxing, aphrodisiac, cooling
TONKA	Bergamot, citronella, clary sage, helichrysum, lavender	Tonic, insecticidal	Tonic, narcotic
VANILLA	Benzoin, sandalwood, spice oils, vetiver	Balsamic	Soothing
VETIVER	Clary sage, jasmine, lavender, patchouli, rose, sandalwood, ylang ylang	Anti-depressant, aphrodisiac	Sedating, strengthening

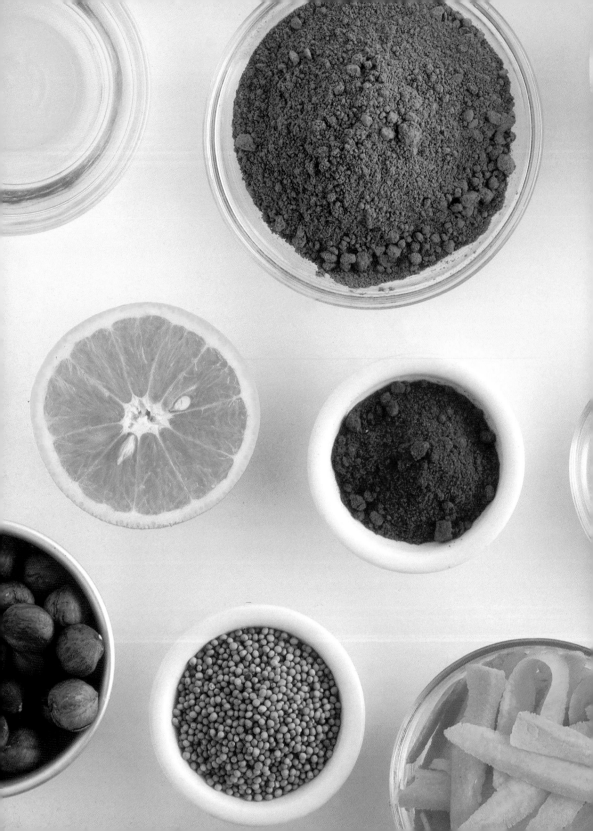

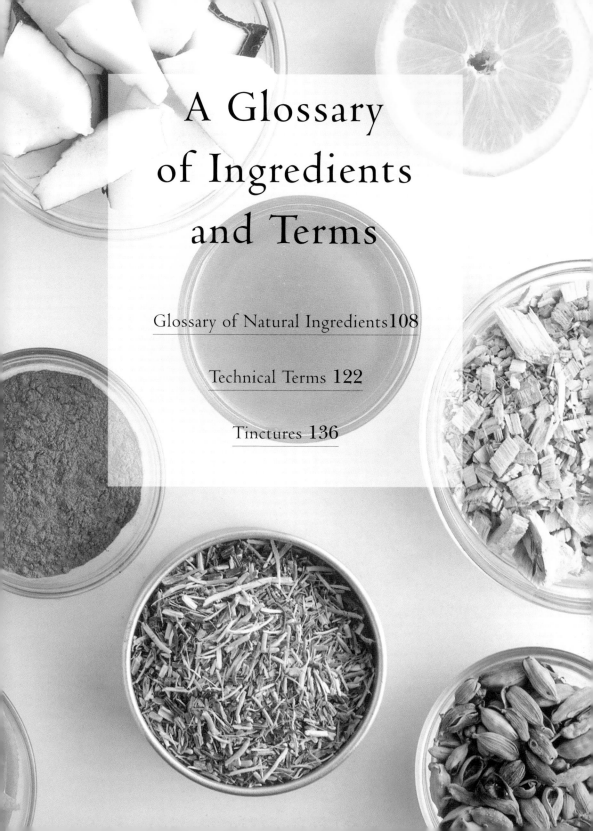

A Glossary of Ingredients and Terms

Glossary of Natural Ingredients

Following is a description of many of the natural ingredients, including herbs and essential oils, used in the recipes in this book. Use this information as a guide to choosing appropriate ingredients when you are making cosmetics for your hair and skin.

Achillea millefolium (yarrow) This herb has astringent, tonic, vulnerary, diaphoretic and diuretic properties. A very good all-round tonic, yarrow is good for poor circulation. It is a very good tonic for female troubles, but it should be avoided internally during pregnancy. Yarrow is excellent for oily or problem skin.

Agnus-castus see *Vitex agnus-castus*.

Allium cepa (onion) The bulb of this plant has antiseptic properties for the skin.

*Althaea officinalis
(marsh mallow)*

Allium sativum (garlic) The bulb of this member of the onion family is an antibiotic and anti-catarrhal, which is used to treat colds, flu, sinusitis, catarrh and any similar infections.

Almond see *Prunus dulcis*.

Aloe vera A mucilage, known as aloe vera juice, is extracted from the plant *Aloe vera* (syn. *A. barbadensis*). It is used externally for its soothing, cooling and anti-irritant properties. It is excellent for treating burns, insect bits and so on. Aloe is an easy plant to grow, and you can simply break off a leaf and use the juice that is produced. Although it is often referred to as a gel, aloe vera juice has more of the consistency of a liquid.

Althaea officinalis (marsh mallow) The herb is a demulcent and healer. Externally, a poultice with slippery elm (*Ulmus rubra*) helps to draw boils and heal ulcers and slow-healing wounds. The root has the same properties as the herb. Marsh mallow tincture is an extract of the herb, produced using alcohol. It has the same properties as the herb.

Angelica archangelica (angelica) The leaves can be used in an infusion. The root is a circulatory stimulant. The plant will also tone the whole system, particularly the digestive system and the lungs. It is also a diuretic and an antiseptic (internally and externally).

Aniseed see *Illicium anisatum*.

Annatto see *Bixa orellana*.

Apium graveolens (celery) Celery seeds are good for itchy and irritated skin.

Apple see *Malus domestica*.

Apple cider vinegar This can be used as an astringent and pH adjuster for both skin and hair. It also contains malic acid, which aids in the removal of dead skin cells. It is a traditional hair rinse when diluted with water. See also *Malus domestica*.

Apricot see *Prunus armeniaca*.

Arctium lappa (burdock) Both the root and leaves of the plant are used. Burdock is an excellent blood purifier for skin disease (taken internally and externally as a wash). As it is antiscorbutic, it may be used to treat boils and skin infections.

Arnica tincture The extraction of the herb *Arnica montana*, produced using water and alcohol, is renowned for its ability to heal bruised skin and ease aching muscles – excellent for sports injuries.

Arrowroot This thickening agent is derived from the rhizomes of a plant of the Marantaceae family.

Astragalus gummifer Tragacanth, a white or reddish gum, is derived from this plant. The gum is used as a thickener and sensitization is possible.

Avena sativa (oats) The cereal nourishes, softens and cleanses the skin. It is excellent to use in facial scrubs and exfoliant preparations, and it is mild enough to be used on sensitive skins.

Avocado see *Persea americana*.

Balm see *Melissa officinalis*.

Balsam of tolu see *Myroxylon balsamum*.

Banana see *Musa acuminata*.

Basil see *Ocimum basilicum*.

Bay See *Laurus nobilis*.

Beeswax Wax produced by the honey-bee (*Apis mellifera*), which contains a mixture of fatty acids and esters. It is used in a range of cosmetics and toiletries as a thickener and emulsifier.

Bergamot see *Citrus bergamia*.

Bilberry see *Vaccinum myrtillus*.

Bixa orellana (annatto, lipstick tree, achiote) The colouring agent from this tree, annatto, contains bixin and several orange-red pigments. It is used as a natural colourant for food and cosmetics.

Black pepper essential oil see *Piper nigrum*.

Blackcurrant see *Ribes nigrum*.

Bladderwrack see *Fucus vesiculosus*.

Boswellia thurifera (frankincense) Olibanum essential oil (or frankincense oil) is distilled from the resin of this tree, which is native to mountainous areas of southern Arabia and India. It has been used for thousands of years as incense, and a few drops placed on an essential oil burner will be uplifting and aid concentration. Its tonifying and rejuvenating properties are of benefit to the mature skins.

Bran The fibrous coating of wheat kernels that is used as an exfoliating agent.

Brassica napus (rape, colza) Rape seed oil is expressed from the seeds of this crop. It is used as a lubricant in soft soaps. It is non-toxic but sensitization is possible.

Brassica nigra (black mustard) Mustard powder, which is made from the ground seeds of this plant, is a stimulant and rubifacient. It increases circulation to a localized area of skin.

Burdock see *Arctium lappa*.

Cajuput see *Melaleuca cajuputi*.

Calendula officinalis (marigold)

Calendula officinalis (marigold) This herb is spasmolytic, anti-haemorrhagic, emmenagogic, vulnerary, styptic and antiseptic. It is a most useful first-aid remedy. Used externally as a wash or cream it is good to heal burns and sores, while the crushed fresh leaf will prevent bleeding and is itself antiseptic. The remedy may also be used externally for varicose veins, ulcers and haemorrhoids, and applied as an eye lotion, when it is a treatment for conjunctivitis. Calendula ointment is used as a soothing and healing treatment for irritated or inflamed skin, for rashes and for eczema. Calendula tincture is an extract of the herb, produced using alcohol, that is antiviral, antibacterial and antifungal. Like the ointment, the tincture can be used to soothe irritated and inflamed skin, and it is an excellent antiseptic healer, which helps to prevent scarring from cuts, burns and boils.

Camellia sinensis (tea) The dried leaf of this familiar shrub is used in cosmetics as a dye and to darken hair colour.

Cananga odorata Ylang ylang essential oil is distilled from the fresh flowers of this tree, which grows in India, Indonesia and the Philippines. The essential oil has a powerful, exotic, floral smell, which has a relaxing effect on the nervous system. It is traditionally used as an aphrodisiac.

Canarium luzonicum Elemi essential oil is distilled from the resin of this tree, which is found in the Philippines. Elemi has a citrus, spicy aroma. It is strongly antiseptic and also has a tonifying and tightening effect. On the skin it has an action similar to myrrh, being cooling and drying. In hair preparations, it balances the secretion of sebum of the scalp.

Candelilla wax A wax obtained from species of the family Euphorbiaceae. It is used in conditioners and lipsticks for its emollient effect.

Capsella bursa-pastoris (shepherd's purse) This is an antihaemorrhagic, urinary, antiseptic, astringent plant, which is useful in the treatment of internal and external bleeding.

Capsicum (pepper) The dried ripe fruit of various species of this shrubby plant is used in external applications in ointments for the treatment of rheumatism. Cayenne pepper, the purest of herbal stimulants, is derived from *C. minimum.* Used externally as a counter-irritant, it is useful in the treatment of rheumatism, arthritis and sciatica. Great care must be taken with the dosage, because this is a very hot remedy indeed.

Cardamom see *Elettaria cardamomum.*

Carrageen A hydrocolloid extracted from an edible, purple seaweed known as Irish moss (*Chondrus crispus*), which is found on rocky shores of the Atlantic in North America and northern Europe. It is used as a thickener in toiletries and food products, and has skin-soothing properties.

Carrot see *Daucus carota.*

Castor oil see *Ricinus communis.*

Cayenne pepper see *Capsicum.*

Cedarwood see *Cedrus libani.*

Cedrus libani (cedar of Lebanon) Cedarwood essential oil is derived from the tree *C. libani* ssp. *atlantica* (Atlas cedar). It has a pleasant, mild, balsamic, woody odour, and it is one of the oldest oils to be produced, having been employed by the ancient Egyptians in the embalming of the dead. It can be used to treat oily skin, oily hair and dandruff.

Chamaemelum nobile (Roman chamomile)

Celery see *Apium graveolens.*

Chamaemelum nobile (syn. *Anthemis nobile,* Roman chamomile) The essential oil is distilled from the herb, which is grown throughout the Mediterranean areas of Europe. The oil is much paler than the oil derived from *Matricaria recutita,* but they have similar, soothing properties, although Roman chamomile is milder and more suitable for children. It is excellent for sensitive skin and eczema.

Chamomile see *Chamaemelum nobile* and *Matricaria recutita.*

Chaste tree see *Vitex agnus-castus.*

Chickweed see *Stellaria media.*

Cider vinegar see Apple cider vinegar.

Cinnamomum camphora (camphor tree) Ho leaf oil is steam-distilled from the leaves of the tree. It has a clean, sweet and floral-woody smell. It is a balancing and calming oil, useful during times of stress.

Cinnamomum zelanicum (cinnamon) The inner bark of this Asian tree is used as a culinary spice and medicinal herb. It is a stimulant and increases the blood flow to a localized area. Cinnamon essential oil is distilled form the inner bark and leaves of the tree. The oil has a powerful, warm, sweetly spicy odour, and it must be well diluted before use because it can be an irritant.

Cinnamon see *Cinnamomum zelanicum.*

Citronella see *Cymbopogon nardus.*

Citrus aurantiifolia (lime) The essential oil is expressed from the unripe peel of the fruit. It has a sharp, fresh smell and has astringent and refreshing properties. This oil may photosensitize the skin and should not be applied before going into the sun.

Citrus aurantium (bitter orange, bigarade) The blossom

of the tree is distilled to make neroli essential oil. Neroli has a delightfully refreshing, powerfully floral smell, and is a classic ingredient of high-quality perfumes. It is a relaxing and uplifting oil, of benefit in treating anxiety, depression and insomnia. In skin care it is useful for dry, mature skin.

Citrus bergamia (bergamot, bergamot orange) Bergamot essential oil is expressed from the peel of the fruit of the tree *C. bergamia*, which is native to Sicily. The oil has an uplifting, sweet, fruity odour. It can be used to make a pleasant, cooling and refreshing massage or bath oil. The oil may photo-sensitize the skin to the sun, causing sunburn, unless the bergaptene has been removed.

Citrus limon (lemon) The fruit of the tree is an astringent and toner, and it decreases the production of sebum. It contains high amounts of vitamin C, and it can be used on the hair to enhance blonde highlights. Lemon essential oil is expressed from the peel of ripe lemons. It has a fresh, sweet smell, truly reminiscent of ripe lemons. It is highly antiseptic and has an astringent effect on the skin. It may be used to treat boils, broken capillaries, greasy skin, herpes and insect bites.

Coriandrum sativum (coriander)

Citrus x paradisi (grapefruit) This refreshing and cooling citrus fruit is high in vitamin C and AHAs. The essential oil is expressed from the peel of the fruit. It has a fresh, sweet, citrus odour and is detoxifying and astringent.

Citrus reticulata (mandarin) The essential oil is expressed from the ripe peel of the fruit. The smell is extremely sweet, and it is a pleasant, safe and refreshing oil to use for adults and children.

Citrus sinensis (orange, sweet orange) Orange essential oil is expressed from the peel of this orange. It is a sweet, refreshing, pleasant oil, with detoxifying properties. Orange flower water, traditionally a by-product of the distillation of orange essential oil, has recently been manufactured by combining neroli essential oil with water, using a dispersing agent. It is specific for mature and dry skin types.

Clary sage see *Salvia sclarea*.

Clove see *Syzygium aromaticum*.

Clover see *Trifolium pratense*.

Cocoa butter see *Theobroma cacao*.

Coconut see *Cocos nucifera*.

Cocos nucifera (coconut) The oil obtained from the pressing of coconuts, the fruit of this palm tree, is used extensively in the production of soaps. It is also an excellent ingredient in skin and hair-care products, when it has an emollient effect. Powdered coconut milk is soothing, softening and moisturizing for the skin. The aroma is more pleasant than that of powdered cow's milk.

Coffea (coffee) Ground coffee is a soothing anti-inflammatory. As a hair rinse, coffee enhances dark highlights.

Coffee see *Coffea*.

Coltsfoot see *Tussilago farfara*.

Comfrey see *Symphytum officinale*.

Commiphora myrrha (myrrh) Myrrh essential oil is distilled from a resin that occurs naturally in the trunks of this small tree, which is native to countries bordering the Red Sea. The oil is an amber-coloured, sticky liquid. It has preserving and antiseptic properties, and it is used to treat infections of the gums, mouth and throat.

Coriander see *Coriandrum sativum*.

Coriandrum sativum (coriander) The essential oil is distilled from the crushed, ripe seeds of this small herb, which is native to southeast Europe. The oil has a fresh, spicy scent. It is a natural deodorant and aphrodisiac.

Corn see *Zea mays*.

Cucumber see *Cucumis sativus*.

Cucumis sativus (cucumber) This salad vegetable has soothing, cooling, refreshing and toning properties. It calms skin irritation.

Cupressus sempervirens (Italian cypress) The essential oil is distilled from the needles and twigs of this evergreen conifer. The smell has a freshness reminiscent of walking through a pine forest. It is an astringent oil that tonifies the venous system and is useful for treating varicose veins, haemorrhoids and broken capillaries.

Cydonia oblonga (quince, common quince) The seed of this small tree is used as a mucilage to thicken cosmetics and as a suspending agent.

Cymbopogon citratus (lemon grass) Lemon grass essential oil is obtained by distillation from this grass. It has a strong, fresh-grass and lemony scent. Lemon grass is a strong anti-bacterial oil, useful for treating problem skin, open pores and acne. It is a good insect repellent.

Cymbopogon martinii Palmarosa essential oil is distilled from this grass, which grows wild in India. It has a pleasant, sweet, rose-like scent and a mildly stimulating effect. It has a regenerative action on the skin.

Cymbopogon nardus (citronella) Citronella essential oil, which has a powerful lemony scent, is distilled from this grass. Its main use is as an effective insect repellent.

Cypress see *Cupressus sempervirens*.

Dandelion see *Taraxacum officinale*.

Daucus carota (carrot) Carrots contain beta-carotene (provitamin A), an antioxidant that protects the skin from free radical damage. Topical application promotes the production of new cells. Eating excess amounts may temporarily discolour the skin. Carrot oil, which is also naturally rich in beta-carotene, is excellent for dry and mature skin.

Equisetum arvense (horsetail)

Echinacea angustifolia (echinacea) The plant is a blood cleanser, which is very useful whenever there is blood poisoning, carbuncles, boils or insect bites. It helps to cleanse morbid matter from the digestive system and encourages lymphatic elimination, so helping to expel poisons, toxins and pus from the body. It may be of benefit in treating fevers and is useful in the treatment of skin conditions.

Elder see *Sambucus nigra*.

Elemi see *Canarium luzonicum*.

Elettaria cardamomum (cardamom) The essential oil that is distilled from this tree, which grows abundantly in India and Sri Lanka, has a warm, spicy, aromatic smell. It has been used in Eastern medicine for more than 3,000 years.

Equisetum arvense (horsetail) The herb contains silica and is useful for strengthening hair and nails.

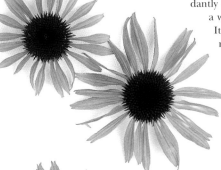

Echinacea angustifolia (echinacea)

Eucalyptus citriodora (lemon-scented gum) This species of eucalyptus has a fresh, sweet, lemony aroma. It is more cooling and refreshing than ordinary eucalyptus, although it shares its antiseptic properties.

Eucalyptus globulus (Tasmanian blue gum) Eucalyptus essential oil is distilled from the leaves of this Australian tree. It is a warming and antiseptic oil, with a strongly camphoraceous and medicinal smell. It is a useful treatment for skin infections and irritation resulting from insect bites.

Euphrasia officinalis (eyebright) As the common name suggests, this makes a very good eyewash if used as a cool, sterile infusion. It is also useful for hayfever.

Evening primrose see *Oenothera biennis.*

Eyebright see *Euphrasia officinalis.*

Fennel see *Foeniculum vulgare.*

Foeniculum vulgare (fennel) Sweet fennel essential oil is steam-distilled from the crushed seeds of *F. vulgare* var. *dulce*, a plant cultivated in Mediterranean Europe. It has a very sweet, fresh smell, which is reminiscent of aniseed. Chewing fennel seeds will freshen the breath. An infusion can also be made to be used as an eyewash to help conjunctivitis.

Fragaria vesca (strawberry) The familiar delicious fruit is said to be able to whiten stained teeth, and it can be added to face masks for cleansing, cooling and astringent properties.

Fucus vesiculosus (bladderwrack) Like many seaweeds, this plant contains many nutritious trace elements, which are often deficient in the modern diet. It is particularly rich in iodine, so it may help those who suffer from an under active thyroid. It is a good dietary supplement.

Garlic see *Allium sativum.*

Geranium see *Pelargonium graveolens.*

Ginger see *Zingiber officinale.*

Glycine max (soya bean) Soya oil is expressed or extracted from soya beans. The oil consists mainly of triglycerides or linoleic and oleic acids. Soya oil is a pale yellow, odourless oil, which is useful for massage or as a base to which essential oils can be added. Sensitization is possible.

Golden rod see *Solidago virgaurea.*

Foeniculum vulgare (fennel)

Golden seal see *Hydrastis canadensis.*

Grapefruit see *Citrus* x *paradisi.*

Grapeseed see *Vitis vinifera.*

Gum A true plant gum is the dried exudate from various plants, obtained when the bark is cut or another injury is sustained. Plant gums are soluble in water and produce very viscous colloidal solutions, sometimes called mucilages.

Gum arabic This fine yellow or white powder, soluble in water, is obtained from some species of *Acacia.* It is also known as gum acacia. It is used as an emulsifying and suspending agent and for the formation of gels. Sensitization is possible.

Hamamelis virginiana (witch hazel) The leaves of the witch hazel have astringent, anti-inflammatory and cooling properties. The name witch hazel also refers to a lotion made from an extract of the leaves in alcohol and water. The lotion is used as a cooling and astringent skin toner and treatment for bruised, inflamed or itchy skin. It is useful in first aid for the treatment of injury and insect bites. It is also an excellent skin toner and cosmetic ingredient for oily or problem skin.

Henna see *Lawsonia inermis.*

Hibiscus The flowers of some species are high in vitamin C and are the source of a strong, deep red dye.

Ho leaf see *Cinnamomum camphora.*

Honey The sweet syrup made by bees is an excellent humectant for moisturizing the skin, and also has antiseptic properties.

Horsetail see *Equisetum arvense.*

Hydrastis canadensis (golden seal) The sacred herb of the Comanche Native Americans. Once called the King of Tonics, it is certainly a wonderful healer for inflammation of the mucous membranes. Externally, it is useful in skin diseases and infections.

Hypericum perforatum (St John's wort) This herb is a marvellous remedy for spinal and nervous problems neuralgia, sciatica and fibrositis, for example. It is antibacterial and can be used for healing, applied locally to burns, wounds and contusions. St John's wort tincture is an extract of the herb, produced through the use of alcohol. It is antibacterial, astringent and healing. St John's wort oil is a macerated oil with a beautiful bright red colour. It is obtained by infusing the herb in vegetable oil (traditionally olive oil), and it is excellent for treating neuralgia, sciatica and any nerve pains as well as burns, sunburn, rashes and shingles. It may cause photosensitivity, so do not apply before exposure to the sun.

Illicium anisatum (aniseed, anise) The essential oil is distilled from the dried and crushed seeds of the tree, which originated in the Near East. The oil has a sweet, fresh smell, and it can be used for cramping, digestive problems and for spasmodic coughs. It has a relatively high toxicity and is best used for only short periods of time.

Hypericum perforatum (St John's wort)

Iris pallida The rhizome of the iris, known as orris root, has been used for many years as a fixative for fragrances, including in pot pourris.

Jasmine see *Jasminum officinale.*

Jasminum officinale (common jasmine) Jasmine absolute is the most uplifting of all the oils. It has an intensely rich and exotic smell, produced from the delicate flowers of the plant. The essential oil can be worn as a delightful perfume, creating a sense of relaxation and enjoyment.

Jojoba see *Simmondsia chinensis.*

Juglans nigra (black walnut) The leaves of the tree can be used to darken the hair.

Juniper see *Juniperus communis.*

Juniperus communis (juniper) The essential oil is distilled from the berries of the juniper tree. It is used in skin preparations to aid oily skin, blocked pores and acne. Juniper oil added to the bath is refreshing and will stimulate the elimination of toxic fluids.

Karite butter see Shea nut butter.

Laurus nobilis (bay, bay laurel, sweet bay) The leaves of this small tree are frequently used in cooking. The medicinal properties are stimulating and cleansing. The essential oil is used mainly for treating sprains and strains.

Lavandula angustifolia (syn. *L. officinalis*; lavender) This herb is soothing, calming and healing for delicate and sensitive skins. Lavender essential oil, with its familiar, sweet fragrance, is one of the most widely used of all essential oils. It has a balancing effect on the nervous system, will relieve headaches and help prevent insomnia. It is very pleasant to use in a massage and in baths. The oil is an excellent antiseptic, is very healing and may be used for burns, wounds, bites, dermatitis and any inflammation of the skin.

Lavender see *Lavandula angustifolia.*

Lawsonia inermis (henna) The powdered leaf of the shrub is traditionally used to dye the skin and hair red.

Lemon see *Citrus limon.*

Lemon balm see *Melissa officinalis.*

Lemon grass see *Cymbopogon citratus.*

Lime see *Citrus aurantiifolia* and *Tilia* x *europaea.*

Malus domestica (apple) Apples are a good source of vitamins C and A as well as containing trace elements of potassium, calcium and magnesium. They also contain malic acid, a 'protein digester', which aids in the removal of dead skin cells. Organic apple juice can be used neat on the skin as an effective toner to remove excess surface oil.

Mandarin see *Citrus reticulata.*

Marigold see *Calendula officinalis* and *Tagetes minuta.*

Marjoram see *Thymus mastichina.*

Marsh mallow see *Althaea officinalis.*

Matricaria recutita (syn. *M. chamomilla*; German chamomile) A most useful remedy, which is excellent externally as a poultice for ulcers, is derived from this medicinal herb, which grows throughout Europe and west Asia. The active volatile oils are best extracted in infusion, but care must be taken not to allow the steam to escape. It may be given with complete safety to nervous children (or adults, for that matter) or to those who suffer from insomnia. It is also good for children's teething troubles. Used externally as a wash or steam bath, it will help clear the skin. It is also a useful eyewash. Chamomile flower water is traditionally a by-product from the distillation of chamomile essential oil, but it is now produced commercially by combining chamomile essential oil with water using a dispersing agent. The flower water is excellent for dry and sensitive skin. Blue chamomile oil, the essential oil that is distilled from the herb, has remarkable anti-inflammatory properties and has a considerable range of uses, including the treatment of allergies, stomach cramps, period pains, insomnia and all kinds of skin irritation and inflammation. See also *Chamaemelum nobile.*

Melaleuca alternifolia Tea tree essential oil is obtained from the leaves of this tree, which is native to Australia. Its excellent germicidal and antifungal properties give it a wide range or uses, including the treatment of colds, flu, herpes, thrush, athlete's foot, warts and other skin infections.

Melaleuca cajuputi (cajuput) An essential oil is distilled from this tree, which grows abundantly in the Philippines and Malaysia. Like that of eucalyptus, the odour is strongly camphoraceous and medicinal. Cajuput essential oil is mainly used in inhalations for respiratory infections, and is especially suitable for relieving symptoms of colds, coughs, sinus infections and sore throats.

Melissa officinalis (lemon balm) This fragrant herb produces one of the most refreshing herbal tisanes. It can often lift the spirits and is a good tonic for the heart, circulation and nervous systems. It is an aid to digestion and helps to relieve tension. The essential oil has a sweet, lemony smell, popular with both children and adults. Melissa essential oil is very uplifting and calming, and itis useful for treating inflamed skin conditions.

Mentha x piperita (peppermint) Peppermint essential oil is distilled from this herb. Peppermint is known for its decongestant, stimulating and refreshing properties. Menthol, which is usually obtained from peppermint, has decongestant and cooling properties.

Mentha x *piperita (peppermint)*

Mentha spicata (syn. *M. viridis*; spearmint) Spearmint makes a refreshing and fragrant infusion, which is cooling for the skin.

Menthol see *Mentha* x *piperita.*

Mullein see *Verbascum thapsus.*

Musa acuminata (banana) The fruit contains high levels of vitamins and minerals, especially potassium. It is humectant and moisturizing.

Mustard see *Brassica nigra.*

Myroxylon balsamum (syn. *M. toluiferum*; tolu balsam tree) The aromatic resin, known as balsam of tolu, of this South American tree is a dark brown fluid that darkens and hardens on ageing. It is used as a conditioner, although some allergic reactions may occur.

Myrrh see *Commiphora myrrha.*

Neroli see *Citrus aurantium.*

Nettle see *Urtica dioica.*

Oats see *Avena sativa*.

Ocimum basilicum (basil) The sweet, spicy, fresh essential oil that is distilled from the herb basil has a calming yet uplifting effect. The oil may irritate sensitive skin if it is not well diluted before use, and it should not be used for prolonged periods.

Oenothera biennis (evening primrose) Pressed oil from the flowers of this plant contains high concentrations of the essential fatty acid gamma linolenic acids, which the human body is unable to make and which must, therefore, be provided in the diet. It is beneficial externally for dry skin and some kinds of eczema.

Olea europaea (common olive) A fixed oil is expressed from the fruit of the tree. Olive oil consists of triglycerides or oleic, linoleic and palmitic acids, and it is used as an emollient and as a soap base. Externally it is soothing, nourishing and lubricant.

Olibanum see *Boswellia thurifera*.

Olive see *Olea europaea*.

Onion see *Allium cepa*.

Orange see *Citrus sinensis*.

Orris root see *Iris pallida*.

Oryza sativa (rice) The grain of this plant is composed essentially of starch. Ground rice can be added to creams and masks to act as an exfoliant. Rice bran oil is extracted from the endosperm of the grain. It is suitable for use in cosmetics and toiletries when low in free fatty acids and all the lipase has been deactivated.

Palm Palm oil is obtained from the seed of the palm tree, cultivated since ancient times. It is used in soaps and as a cosmetic ingredient for its lubricant properties. It has no known toxicity. Palm kernel oil is an edible fat obtained from palm kernels to make soap. It is also used as an ingredient in cosmetics for its emollient properties. It, too, has no known toxicity.

Palmarosa see *Cymbopogon martinii*.

Parsley see *Petroselinum crispum*.

Patchouli see *Pogostemon cablin*.

Pelargonium graveolens (rose geranium, sweet-scented geranium) Geranium essential oil is produced from the leaves of this species. It is a cooling and calming oil, useful for treating anxiety and tension. It has a balancing effect on the skin, making it suitable for dry, oily or problem skin, and it is a very pleasant oil to use in the bath or as a massage oil.

Peppermint see *Mentha* x *piperita*.

Persea americana (syn. *P. gratissima*; avocado pear) The fruit of the tree is naturally rich in unsaturated oils, which hydrate, nourish and moisturize the skin. Avocado oil, which is expressed from the flesh of the avocado pear, is dark green. It is an excellent emollient and natural colourant, and it contains oleic, linoleic and palmitic acids.

Petroselinum crispum (parsley) This popular culinary herb also soothes, cleanses and heals the skin, and it is used when the skin is irritated and inflamed. It contains high levels of vitamins C and A.

Pine see *Pinus sylvestris*.

Pinus sylvestris (Scots pine) Pine essential oil is distilled from the needles and wood chippings of this tree. It has a refreshing, sweet, woody smell, and is an effective antiseptic and deodorant.

Piper nigrum (black pepper) The essential oil is produced by steam distillation of the dried, crushed fruits of this climbing plant, which is grown mainly in Indonesia and India. It is a hot, dry, spicy oil, with a deeply warming effect, and it is useful for relieving muscular aches and pains and for its detoxifying properties. Black pepper oil must be well diluted before it is applied to the skin.

Pogostemon cablin (syn. *P. patchouly*) Patchouli essential oil is distilled from the dried leaves of this small plant. It has a persistent, dry-wood smell and is used in perfumery for its fixative properties. Patchouli is claimed to be an aphrodisiac, and it may be used in skin care to reduce scarring and to treat oily and problem skin.

Potato see *Solanum tuberosum*.

Prunus armeniaca (apricot) Apricot kernel oil, also known as peach kernel oil, is the oil expressed from the kernels of the fruit of this tree.

Prunus dulcis (almond) Sweet almond oil, a fixed oil, is expressed from the kernels of varieties of *P. dulcis*. It is a light, odourless oil, with soothing, nourishing and skin-conditioning properties. It is a popular massage base oil, and it is also used as an emollient in many skin-care creams and lotions. Sensitization is possible. Almond meal, the residue that is left after almond oil has been expressed, is an excellent exfoliant. Ground almonds, too, make a very useful exfoliant.

Quassia amara Quassia chips are derived from the bark of this tree and of *Picrasma excelsa*, which are native to South America. The chips have an extremely bitter taste, but a hair rinse made from quassia chips can be used as an effective treatment for head lice.

Ribes nigrum (blackcurrant)

Quillaja saponaria (soap-bark tree) The inner dried bark of this tree is known as soap bark, quillaja or quillay. Extracts are used as a natural detergent and natural foaming agent. Quillaja is a saponin, and it is used in shampoos, shower gels and creams and also as a foam stabilizer in soft drinks. It is non-toxic to mammals but is toxic to crustaceans, and its use is, therefore, of environmental concern.

Quince see *Cydonia oblonga*.

Rape see *Brassica napus*.

Raspberry see *Rubus idaeus*.

Rheum x hybridum (syn. *R.* x *culturom*; rhubarb) This edible garden plant is used medicinally as an astringent and purgative. Externally, it may be used to lighten the hair. The leaves should not be eaten.

Rhubarb see *Rheum* x *hybridum*.

Ribes nigrum (blackcurrant) The leaves of the shrub are used as an astringent to decrease the production of sweat and to reduce pore size.

Rice see *Oryza sativa*.

Ricinus communis (castor oil plant) The thick, colourless oil that is extracted from the plant provides a protective, waterproof coating to both the skin and hair.

Rosa (rose) Pink and red rose buds may be used medicinally for their cooling and soothing action. They may be used as an infusion for itchy, inflamed or sunburned skin. Hips, the fruits or berries from wild rose bushes, notably *R. canina* (dog rose) and *R. gallica* (French rose), which contain high concentrations of vitamin C, make a pleasant infusion for drinking on their own or combined with hibiscus. Rose hip oil, which is extracted from the hips of *R. canina*, is claimed to be of use in treating scar tissue. Rose water was traditionally a by-product of the

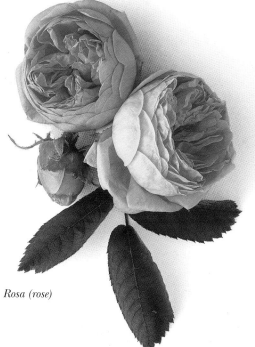

Rosa (rose)

117

steam-distillation of rose essential oil, but it is now man-ufactured commercially by combining rose absolute with water, using a dispersing agent. A cooling, anti-inflammatory lotion for itchy, inflamed or reddened skin, it also helps to maintain the skin's natural water balance. It is a good skin toner with a pleasant fragrance and is suitable for any skin type. Rose essential oil is an exquisite oil produced from *R.* x *damascena* var. *semperflo-rens* (damask rose) and *R.* x *cen-tifolia* (Provence rose, cabbage rose). It is a cooling and sooth-ing oil, which is excellent for treating stress-related conditions and menstrual problems, including PMT. It is beneficial for dry, inflamed and mature skins. Rose absolute is pro-duced by solvent extraction, while the very cost-ly true rose oil is steam-distilled.

Rose see *Rosa*.

Rosemary see *Rosmarinus officinalis*

Rosmarinus officinalis (rosemary) The herb is found growing wild throughout the Mediterranean countries, and it has been used for centuries as a culinary and medicinal herb. The volatile oils have strong antiseptic properties. It makes an excellent rinse for the hair. Rosemary essential oil is refreshing and stimulating. It is excellent for hair and scalp problems, including hair loss and dandruff.

Rubus idaeus (raspberry) The leaves of this shrub are anti-spasmodic, astringent and stimulant. It is good for sore throats and bleeding gums.

Sage see *Salvia officinalis*.

St John's wort see *Hypericum perforatum*.

Salvia officinalis (common sage) This herb, native to countries around the north Mediterranean, is a natural antibiotic, useful as a gargle in sore throats. It is an anti-septic to the skin and darkens the hair. It is also useful in the treatment of dandruff. Sage relieves excessive sweat-ing. Do not take during pregnancy. Sage essential oil is distilled from the herb. It has a fresh, herbaceous and camphoraceous smell. It is a strongly simulating oil,

Sambucus nigra (elder)

which will relieve muscular aches and pains, reduce excessive sweating and is tra-ditionally used in mouthwashes for gum and mouth infections.

Salvia sclarea (clary sage) The essential oil derived from this herb has a bitter-sweet, herby odour. It has a soothing and sedating effect, while at the same time strengthening the nervous system. It is useful for treating stress, anxiety and depression and for hasten-ing convalescence.

Sambucus nigra (elder) Its somewhat astringent property has made elderflower water a favourite wash for greasy or problem skin. A steam facial will do much to clear blackheads.

Sandalwood see *Santalum album*.

Santalum album (sandalwood) Sandalwood essential oil is distilled from the wood of the tree. It has long been regarded as having aphrodisiac properties, and it makes a popular massage oil. Sandalwood is par-ticularly beneficial for dry skin.

Saponaria officinalis (soapwort) Infusions of soapwort have been used as a cleanser for the hair and skin for cen-turies.

Seaweed A number of different seaweeds, most notably bladderwrack (*Fucus vesiculosus*), carrageen and kelp, have a use in cosmetics and toiletries. Seaweed is a rich natural source of many minerals, vitamins and trace ele-ments, and they have a long history of use in external applications as cleansing, detoxifying, toning and condi-tioning agents.

Shea nut butter (also known as karite butter) A natural fat obtained from the fruit of the tree *Butyrospermum parkii*. It has no known toxicity.

Shepherd's purse see *Capsella bursa-pastoris*.

Simmondsia chinensis (jojoba) Jojoba oil is a semi-liquid, oil-like wax obtained from the leaves of this shrub. It has excellent emollient properties.

Slippery elm see *Ulmus rubra.*

Soap bark see *Quillaja saponaria.*

Soapwort see *Saponaria officinalis.*

Solanum tuberosum (potato) Potatoes are high in vitamin C. They will reduce puffiness around the eyes if sliced and placed on the eyes.

Solidago virgaurea (golden rod) This herb has astringent and toning properties.

Soya see *Glycine max.*

Spearmint see *Mentha spicata.*

Stellaria media (chickweed) This common garden weed has a cooling action on the body tissues and is useful for external inflammation – as a poultice for boils, for example, or in an ointment for itching, eczema and skin rashes.

Strawberry see *Fragaria vesca.*

Symphytum officinale (comfrey) The old country name, 'knitbone', tells of the great healing potential of this herb. Used externally as a compress, it helps fractured bones to mend and cuts, ulcers and bruises to heal with minimal scar formation. It is very nutritious. Comfrey tincture is an alcoholic extraction that provides the same properties as the herb.

Syzygium aromaticum (syn. *Eugenia caryophyllus*; clove) The essential oil is obtained by distillation of the flower-buds of the evergreen clove tree, which originated in the Moluccas. It has a strongly stimulating effect and also has pain-relieving properties, which are especially valuable for relieving toothache. It is a very antiseptic oil and is useful as a room fumigant. Clove oil may irritate the skin and must be well diluted before use.

Tagetes minuta (syn. *T. glandulifera*) Tagetes essential oil is distilled from a type of marigold. It has a bright orange-green colour and sweet, herbaceous smell. It is particularly useful for treating foot problems such as hardened skin, corns and verrucas. This oil may photosensitize the skin and should not be applied before going into the sun.

Taraxacum officinale (dandelion) Were the dandelion a rare plant, its medicinal qualities would make it worth a fortune. The leaves are strongly diuretic (hence its French name, *pis-en-lit*) and rich in potassium, which means that no potassium supplement is required, as is the case with most drug diuretics. It is, therefore, very useful in any condition in which there is fluid retention. It is also a blood purifier and spring tonic. Its cleansing properties make it a useful herb for treating many skin problems, such as acne.

Tea see *Camellia sinensis.*

Tea tree see *Melaleuca alternifolia.*

Theobroma cacao (cacao, chocolate nut tree) Cocoa butter is the fat that is obtained from the roasted seeds of the cocoa bean, the fruit of this tree. The butter contains stearic, palmitic and oleic acids, and it is used as an emollient and conditioning agent.

Thuja occidentalis Thuja tincture is a strong anti-viral remedy derived from this tree. Apply to warts and verrucas, but apply sparingly to the skin.

Thyme see *Thymus vulgaris.*

Thymus vulgaris (thyme)

Thymus mastichina (marjoram) The essential oil is steam-distilled form the dried leaves and flowering tops of this well-known herb. It is a warming and relaxing oil, useful for treating stress, anxiety and insomnia. It is also used to relieve aching muscles, rheumatism, strains and period pains.

Thymus vulgaris (thyme) An infusion of the herb is fragrant as well as being antiviral, antifungal and antibacterial. It is traditionally used to add shine and strength to dark hair. Thyme essential oil is distilled from the herb. It is a warming and stimulating oil that will relieve muscular pain. It is used to treat many kinds of infections – for example, skin, respiratory and urinary – because it is strongly antimicrobial and also strengthens the immune response. The oil must be well diluted before use because it may irritate sensitive skin.

Tilia x **europaea** (lime) A very soothing remedy is made from the flowers of the tree. It may be used for its soothing properties both internally and externally.

Tragacanth see *Astragalus gummifer*.

Trifolium pratense (red clover) Taken internally, the flowers purify the blood and can aid many skin conditions. It is rich in minerals.

Tussilago farfara (coltsfoot) This plant's generic name comes from the Latin word meaning 'to cough'. It is one

Urtica dioica (nettle)

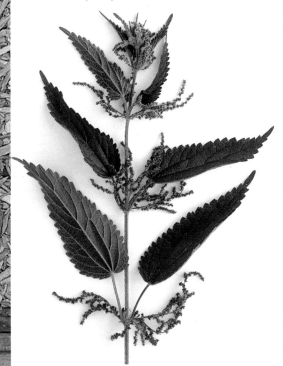

Rubus idaeus (raspberry)

of nature's great pulmonary remedies, useful in all chest complaints. Both flowers and leaves are used, and the plant is rich in magnesium, so it may also help in skin complaints.

Ulmus rubra (syn. *U. fulva*; slippery elm) This tree provides one of nature's most useful remedies. Slippery elm is nutritious, demulcent and healing, with a very gentle action. Applied externally as a poultice, it is wonderfully soothing and drawing for injured or inflamed parts. It helps to speed healing, when it may be combined with comfrey (*Symphytum officinale*), marshmallow (*Althea officinalis*) and marigold (*Calendula officinalis*).

Urtica dioica (stinging nettle) Rich in minerals, this is one of nature's finest spring tonics (especially the new green shoots). It is excellent for anaemia and will slough off the clogging foods of winter, reviving the system. It can be eaten as food either in soups or as a vegetable. It is useful externally as a wash for a dry, flaking scalp.

Vaccinum myrtillus (bilberry, whinberry, whortleberry) The fruits of this shrub contain fruit acids that can be used to whiten the teeth.

Valerian see *Valeriana officinalis*.

Verbascum thapsus (mullein) Mullein oil is a macerated oil made with the herb mullein and vegetable oil. It is used to treat earache and blocked ears.

Vervain see *Verbena officinalis*.

Vetiver see *Vetiveria zizanoides*.

Vetiveria zizanoides (vetiver) Vetiver essential oil is distilled from the roots of this scented grass, which grown mainly in India and Indonesia. It has a sweet, woody and earthy smell and astringent properties. It may be used to treat oily skin, acne and weeping skin conditions.

Vitex agnus-castus (agnus-castus, chaste tree) The berries are used to produce agnus-castus, which has a reputation as a normalizer of pituitary function. It is useful in cases of PMT, menstrual irregularity and whenever male or female hormonal imbalance is involved. It can be used to treat periodic skin problems.

Vitis vinifera (common grape vine) Grapeseed oil, which comes from the vine, is quickly and deeply absorbed by the skin, making it suitable for light massage of delicate or oily skin. It is odourless and almost colourless, and is, therefore, an ideal base to which essential oils can be added.

Walnut see *Juglans nigra.*

Wheatgerm oil This heavy, rich oil is a natural source of vitamin E. Used alone, it is rather a heavy oil with a distinctive odour; for massage, it can be combined with a lighter oil, such as almond oil, or it can be used to help avoid stretch marks during pregnancy.

Whinberry, whortleberry see *Vaccinum myrtillus.*

Witch hazel see *Hamamelis virginiana.*

Yarrow see *Achillea millefolium.*

Ylang ylang see *Cananga odorata.*

Yogurt Produced by the action of bacteria on milk, yogurt cleanses and conditions the skin and is readily absorbed. It contains lactic acid, which is thought to stimulate cell production. It is a useful treatment for thrush (*Candida albicans*) when applied locally.

Zea mays (maize, sweet corn) Cornstarch (cornflour) is the milled powder derived from maize. The size of the particles makes it an excellent exfoliant, although sensitization is possible. Corn oil, which is also obtained from maize, is used as an emollient and naturally contains tocopherols and lecithin, which are excellent for moisturizing; again, sensitization is possible. Corn silk, which is obtained from the cobs of maize, is a soothing demulcent for the urinary system and is especially useful for the burning pains of cystitis and other urinary system infections.

Zingiber officinale (ginger) The root of this plant, a native to the tropical coastal regions of India, is a very good circulatory stimulant. Ginger essential oil is a deeply warming oil, which will help to stimulate the circulation to an area. It may be used to treat rheumatism, sprains and strains.

Technical Terms

Increasingly, manufacturers of cosmetics are obliged to list all the ingredients they use on their product packaging. This glossary includes explanations of many of the chemical ingredients of commercially prepared cosmetics as well as definitions of many chemical terms to help you interpret this information.

Absolute An aromatic, volatile substance obtained by solvent extraction from a single botanical species – for example rose absolute and jasmine absolute. None of the solvent should remain after the process is complete, when absolutes may be used like essential oils.

Acetamide MEA A synthetic raw material used as a hair conditioner and solvent. It has low toxicity to the skin and eyes.

Acetic acid An acid in vinegar and used as a preservative in foods and a solvent for gums and volatile oils.

Acetone A solvent used mainly in nail varnishes and nail polish removers. It is an irritant, and its use in cosmetics has been banned or restricted in many countries.

Acid colours Synthetic dyes used to colour food, cosmetics and toiletries. The list of allowable acid colours has been reduced dramatically in recent years because they are highly irritant.

Acids Substances that, when added to water, liberate hydrogen as an ion. They also react with bases to form salts. Acids have a low pH value (pH7 being neutral). Note that strong acids can be highly irritant; weak acids are beneficial to the skin, which is naturally slightly acidic.

Acne Although this is the commonest skin complaint, affecting an estimated 80 per cent of teenagers at any one time, its causes are still not fully understood. It affects both females and males in the same numbers, although the condition is usually more severe in young males and hence more noticeable.

Active ingredients The ingredients contained in any formula that give the desired physiological effect – for example, the component in a moisturizing cream that improves the moisture content of the skin.

Alkalis Substances with a pH above 7 that are often used as neutralizers in cosmetics and toiletries. Strongly alkaline substances are corrosive – for example, caustic soda.

Alkaloids Plant substances with an organic nitrogen base that often have pharmacological properties. For example, valerianine is an alkaloid present in the herb valerian.

Alkyloamides A common family of ingredients, including Cocamide DEA, MEA, MIPA or PEG, used in shampoos, bubble baths and liquid hand and body cleansers. They are employed for thickening, gelling, emulsifying and solubilizing. The major drawback with alkyloamides is that they can be contaminated with nitrosamines during manufacture of the product. Nitrosamines are suspected animal carcinogens. Correct formulation and the use of a reputable supplier will help eliminate the risk.

Allantoin A product that is synthetically produced by the oxidation of uric acid and found naturally in comfrey root and uva ursi. Used as a humectant, conditioner and detoxicant, it has soothing and anti-irritant properties.

Allergy A hypersensitive reaction to specific substances that develops in some people. It is characterized by an irritation such as redness or itching.

Aluminosilicates Silicates containing aluminium, which are a major compound found in many clays, such as kaolin or bentonite.

Ambergris A waxy substance, secreted by sperm whales. It is used as a fixative in perfumery.

Amino acids Group of compounds containing both the carboxyl (COOH) and the amino (NH2) groups. They are the building blocks of proteins and are crucial to the maintenance of the body. Essential amino acids – for example, histidine, leucine and lysine – cannot be manufactured by the body and must be supplied in the diet. Non-essential amino acids – arginine, cystine and taurine, for example – are manufactured by the body.

Ammonium laureth sulphate A synthetic detergent that is used extensively as the primary surfactant in shampoos as a foaming and cleansing agent. Some problems can arise from the ethoxylated detergents. See also Ethoxylate.

Ammonium lauryl sulphate The ammonium salt of sulphated lauryl alcohol, which is used as a foaming and cleansing agent. The absence of any ethoxylation makes it slightly less mild than ammonium laureth sulphate but excludes the problems associated with ethoxylation. See also Ethoxylate.

Ammonium pareth-25 sulphate An anionic surfactant used for its foaming and cleansing properties. It is an inexpensive detergent that, if used in high concentrates, can cause eye and skin irritation.

Amphoteric surfactant See Surfactant.

Amygdalin A glucoside found in the kernels of most fruit belonging to the Rosaceae family, particularly bitter almonds. It is used widely as a flavouring material in the form of essence of bitter almonds. Although harmless in small doses in its natural form, it becomes toxic when distilled, hence the toxicity of bitter almond oil.

Anionic surfactant See Surfactant.

Antibacterial Any agent or process that inhibits the growth and reproduction of bacteria. Preservatives have antibacterial properties, and are used to protect products from degradation. Many essential oils are antibacterial.

Antioxidants Substances that prevent the formation of free radicals, which can cause the oxidative deterioration that causes rancidity in oils or fats and also premature ageing. Examples of natural antioxidants include vitamins A, C and E.

Antiperspirants Substances that inhibit perspiration and cause blocking of the skin's pores. They are generally based on either aluminium zirconin or zinc salts.

Arachidonic acid An essential fatty acid that is found in beeswax and some natural oils.

Astringents Products that cause a tightening and contraction of the skin tissues, generally used to tone skin and close pores.

Azulene An anti-inflammatory component found in chamomile flowers. Chamazulene is the blue component that gives chamomile oil its distinctive colour.

Barrier cream A cream that provides a barrier when applied to the skin and produces a protective coating. Generally, barrier creams are quite oily products or contain lanolin.

Bentonite A form of clay that swells in the presence of water to give a gel. It is used as a thickening agent and is considered non-toxic.

Benzaldehyde The major component of bitter almond oil. It is often synthesized for its almond fragrance and is used in cosmetics and toiletries. It can produce allergic reactions in sensitive individuals.

Benzalkonium chloride A cationic surfactant used in conditioners and shampoos for conditioning the hair and as an anti-dandruff ingredient. It has bactericidal activity and is also used in mouthwashes and aftershave preparations. It can be a severe irritant to the eyes and skin if used in high concentrations.

Benzene A petrochemical used as a solvent and manufacturing agent in lacquers, varnishes and cosmetics. Highly toxic in even minute proportions, it has known carcinogenic activity.

Benzoic acid A white powder that is used as an anti-microbial agent both in food products and in toiletries. It is slightly toxic and can cause skin irritations.

Benzoin A resin obtained from various *Styrax* species, which has a warming odour. It is used as a fixative, preservative and antioxidant and for its skin-healing properties. In its natural state it is solid, so it is dissolved in a solvent for ease of use. It is good for dry, cracked or chapped skin and also has antiseptic properties. It is not to be taken internally.

Benzophenones These are used as fixatives in perfumes. Benzophenone-3 absorbs ultra-violet light and is therefore used as a sunscreen agent, especially for UVA protection. Allergic reactions can occur.

Benzyl alcohol A colourless liquid that is used as a bactericide and solvent. It has an anaesthetizing action, and high concentrations can cause irritations.

Betaines Derivatives of trimethyl glydine that occur chiefly in plants. Surfactants, such as coco betaine, are formed by linking them to a fatty acid chain. They are used to decrease the irritancy potential of some anionic surfactants, such as sodium laureth sulphate. They have no known toxicity.

Bha (butylated hydroxanisole) A white, waxy solid that is used as an antioxidant to prevent oxidative deterioration of oils and fats. It is synthetic.

Bht (butylated hydroxytoluene) A synthetic antioxidant, which can cause sensitization.

Borax (sodium borate) A mild alkali that is used in cosmetics and toiletries as a water softener, preservative and texturizer. When making simple creams and lotions it may be safely used in combination with beeswax as an emulsifier. Not toxic externally, there is some toxicity internally and it should not be applied to broken skin. Keep out of reach of children.

Botanical extract An extract of herbs and plants. The extracting solvent can be water, oil, alcohol or any synthetic solvent such as propylene glycol.

2-bromo-2 nitropropane 1-3 diol An antimicrobial agent, active against bacteria and fungi. It can react with secondary amines and form nitrosamines, which are known carcinogens. Used at high levels it can cause irritation.

Butyl paraben Butyl p-hydroxybenzoate. See Parabens.

Calamine A pink powder made of zinc oxide with a small amount of ferric oxide. It is a traditional mixture used for relieving itchy skin and rashes. It is not generally considered to be toxic.

Calcium carbonate Commonly known as chalk, a naturally occurring calcium salt found in limestone, coral and marble. It is used as an abrasive agent in toothpastes and face washes and also as a whitener and neutralizer in cosmetics. It has no known toxicity.

Candida albicans A yeast that causes thrush and, in more severe cases, symptoms affecting the whole body. Recent studies have shown that tea tree oil can be very effective at treating this infection locally.

Capric acid A fatty acid that is used as an emollient in creams. It occurs as glycerides in the milk of goats and cows, and in coconut and palm oil.

Caramel A concentrated solution of heated sugar that can be used as a natural colouring agent.

Carbomer-934 A polymer of acrylic acid that is used as a thickener. It is considered to be of essentially low toxicity.

Carboxymethyl hydroxycellulose A derivative of cellulose that has been chemically modified for use as a thickener and stabilizer in creams, lotions and ice cream. It is considered non-toxic externally, although some toxicity is reported internally.

Carmine A red substance used as a dye and colourant, obtained from the female cochineal insect.

Carotene One of the most important colouring matters of green leaves. It is found in all plants and in many animal tissues. Beta-carotene (provitamin A) is the yellow colouring matter of carrots and egg yolk. It is used as a natural colourant in cosmetics.

Casein A protein found in the milk of mammals. It is used as a hair thickener and conditioner and as an emulsifier. It has no known toxicity.

Cationic surfactant See Surfactant.

Caustic soda (sodium hydroxide) A common reagent that is widely used in the manufacture of soap.

Cellulose gum A synthetic gum, of which the starting material is cellulose, used as a thickener and stabilizer.

Ceteareth-5 Cetearyl alcohol, which has been rendered soluble in water by condensing it with ethylene oxide. Used as a thickener and emulsifier, it has no known toxicity.

Cetearyl alcohol Also known as cetyl stearyl alcohol or emulsifying wax, this is a mixture of cetyl and stearyl alcohols, which may be animal, vegetable or petrochemical derived. It is used as an emulsifier, emollient and thickener and is excellent for use in homemade creams and conditioners. It has no known toxicity.

Cetrimonium chloride A cationic surfactant, which is a quaternary ammonium salt. It is used in conditioners and also as an antiseptic and preservative. Concentrated solutions can irritate the skin, and it is toxic internally.

Cetyl alcohol An alcohol consisting of mainly n-hexadecanol. It is used as a thickener and emulsifier. See also Cetearyl alcohol.

Chelatory agent A substance that binds minerals to itself. In cosmetic manufacture it refers to chemicals that mop up free ions, such as metals, in formulae and inhibit them from causing deterioration of the product.

TECHNICAL TERMS

Chloromethyl isothiarzolinone One of the components of Kathon GG, which is the trade name for a commonly used preservative. Its popularity is due to its effectiveness at very low concentrations. Skin sensitization is possible.

Chlorophyll The green pigment of plants that is essential for photosynthesis. It is used as a natural colourant.

Chloroxylenol An antimicrobial agent used in treatment shampoos and antiseptic lotions. It is apparently non-irritant at low dilutions of less than 5 per cent.

Citric acid A component of citrus fruits used as a pH modifier in cosmetics and foods. It has no known toxicity.

Clay A natural aluminosilicate – that is, a compound based on aluminium and silicon and oxygen. It is used in face masks because of its absorbing, cleansing ability and also as a thickener in some shampoo ingredients.

Coal tar Tar obtained during the distillation of coal. It is used as an anti-dandruff ingredient. It can cause dermatitis on the skin.

Cocamide DEA An unchanged (non-ionic) surfactant, derived from chemically modified coconut oil.

Cocamidopropyl betaine Properly called cocamido-propyl dimethyl glycine, this member of the betaine family is used as a mild foaming and cleansing agent to reduce the irritancy of harsher surfactants in shampoos.

Cocobetaine An amphoteric surfactant, which is based on chemical modifications to coconut oil. It is included in shampoos and cleansing rinses and, used correctly, will help render certain other surfactants more mild.

Cocotrimonium chloride An antionic surfactant used as a hair conditioner. It can be an irritant to the eyes.

Coemulisifiers Secondary emulsifiers that improve the stability of emulsion systems.

Collagen The most abundant protein in the body, containing mainly glycerine, hydroxyproline and prioline. It is found in all connective tissues – for example, skin, cartilage, tendons, ligaments. When the collagen in the skin deteriorates, due to ageing or overexposure to the sun, the appearance of the skin is affected by wrinkles. It is sometimes used in cosmetics and toiletries, although there is no evidence that external application is effective.

Concrète The product obtained from solvent extraction of an aromatic material. The solvent is generally evaporated off to leave behind the absolute and the concrète.

Contact dermatitis A condition in which the skin has become damaged through topical contact with chemicals. Two types exist: primary irritation, which occurs at the time of contact and can cause itchy swelling and redness, and allergic sensitization, in which symptoms arise after several exposures to the chemical.

Coupling agent A material used to increase the solubility of one ingredient in another.

Cream The source of highly concentrated proteins, which are readily absorbed by the skin.

D & C colours D stands for Drugs and C for Cosmetics. It is an American system for classifying the areas in which these various colours can be used.

DEA lauryl sulphate Diethanolamine salt of lauryl sulphate, used as a foaming and cleansing agent. It may be irritant in concentration.

Decyl alcohol An anti-foam agent, fixative, lubricant and emollient. It occurs naturally in some plant oils but is commercially extracted from coconut oil or paraffin. It has no known toxicity.

Dimethicone Dimethicone copolyol, a polymer based on silicone, which is used as a conditioner in hair care products and as a skin protectant. It has a tendency to build up on the hair shaft, eventually making the hair appear dull and is not, therefore, currently favoured. It is not considered toxic.

Deodorant Any product that masks the odour produced by the action of bacteria or sweat. Unlike an antiperspirant, a deodorant does not interfere with the production of sweat.

Depilatory A preparation designed to aid hair removal. This may be chemical (as in hair-dissolving creams) or mechanical, for example a wax.

Detergent A chemical that is used as a cleansing agent and unlike soap does not derive directly from fats and oils. Detergents modify the interface between two surfaces (see Surfactant). They may derive from petroleum (most household detergents) or vegetable oil.

125

Dimethyl stearamine See Surfactant.

Dioctyl sodium sulfosuccinate Used as a dispersing agent and solubilizer. It is non-irritant in dilution.

Dipentene Another name for limonene.

Dipropylene glycol See Propylene glycol.

Disodium EDTA A compound used as an antioxidant, preservative and chelating agent to form complexes with elements and stop any catalytic reactions from occurring. It is not generally considered to be toxic externally, although sensitization is possible.

Disodium monococamido sulfosuccinate See Dioctyl sodium sulfosuccinate.

Disodium phosphate See Sodium phosphate.

DMDM hydantoin A water-soluble preservative. It can be toxic at a high level, but used within the guidelines is essentially safe. See also Disodium EDTA.

EDTA Ethylene diamine tetra acetic acid, used as a chelating agent in shampoos and also as an antioxidant. It is chemically synthesised. See also Disodium EDTA.

Elastin A protein of elastic tissue, ligaments and arterial wall. It is structurally related to collagen.

Electrolyte A substance that undergoes partial or complete dissociation into ions in solution. Electrolytes are important in cosmetics and toiletries because they can affect viscosity and other properties of the product. Salt, for example, is a common electrolyte used to thicken some shampoos.

Emollient Any substance that prevents water loss from the skin. Most natural oils perform this function.

Emulsifier A substance that holds oil in water or water in oil. Examples include borax, beeswax and cetearyl alcohol. Emulsifiers are necessary in the manufacture of creams and lotions.

Emulsifying wax A wax used to prepare stable emulsions such as creams and lotions. See also Cetearyl alcohol.

Emulsion A mixture of two incompatible substances. Most creams on the cosmetic market are emulsions consisting of oil-soluble ingredients mixed with water-soluble ingredients by the use of emulsifiers.

Enzyme A biological catalyst that acts to speed up chemical reactions. Digestive enzymes are necessary for the breakdown of protein, carbohydrates and fats – for example, pancreatin, pepsin.

Epsom salts Magnesium sulphate used as a purgative and in bath salts used for detoxifying and relaxation.

Essential oil The odorous, volatile product of a known botanical origin. Most essential oils are produced by steam distillation, although several are mechanically expressed. They are used therapeutically in aromatherapy. When using essential oils at home, it is important to know the plant species, origin, chemotype and the method of extraction of the oil if you are looking for a therapeutic benefit. See also Absolute.

Essential fatty acid A fatty acid that must be supplied in the diet as the body cannot produce it itself. They include linoleic, linolenic and arachidonic acids. The first two are found in evening primrose oil and the latter in beeswax.

Ester A derivative of an acid. Many esters have fruity smells and are used in artificial fruit essences.

Ethanol Alcohol is manufactured by the fermentation of sugar, starch and other carbohydrates. Ethanol, or ethyl alcohol, used in cosmetic formulation such as perfumes and aftershaves is usually denatured by the addition of an unpleasant-tasting chemical to stop consumption.

Ethanolamine A component manufactured by heating ethylene oxide under pressure with concentrated aqueous ammonia. They form soaps with fatty acids. They are used for pH control or, when linked to fatty acids, as solubilizers and thickeners. The di- and tri-ethanolamines are able to form highly toxic nitrosamines under certain conditions and so their manufacture must be carefully monitored. Can be irritant in high concentrations.

Ethoxylate A substance that has had ethylene oxide added to render it more water soluble. There is some concern about the impact of the ethoxylation process on the environment because of the presence of 1,4 Dioxane, a by-product of the process and a suspected carcinogen.

Ethyl parabens See Parabens.

Eucalyptol Also known as 1,8 Cineole. The chief component of the essential oil of *Eucalyptus globulus.*

Eugenol The chief constituent of clove oil but also found in cinnamon oil and bay oil. It has excellent antiseptic properties.

Exfoliate To remove surface layers of the skin, especially dead skin cells, generally by the use of an abrasive agent.

Expression Describes the technique used for extracting essential oils from citrus products. See also Essential oil.

Fat A greasy solid that is an ester of fatty acids and glycerol. Fats can be used in the soap-making process, and glycerol is generally a by-product.

Fatty acid A monobasic acid containing only the chemicals carbon, hydrogen and oxygen. Found in vegetable and animal fats, they are important for maintaining a healthy skin and are excellent emollients.

Fatty acid alkanolamides See Ethanolamine.

F D & C colours Refers to colours that are permitted in the USA in food, drugs and cosmetics.

Fixative A material that helps to slow the rate of evaporation of components of perfume formulations, thereby making the fragrance last longer. Certain essential oils, for example sandalwood, have fixative properties.

Filtration The process of separating a solid from a liquid or gas by the use of a membrane that will allow only the liquid to pass through.

Fixed oil A fixed oil is chemically the same as a fat, but is generally liquid. Examples include almond oil, apricot kernel oil and grapeseed oil.

Fluoride This inorganic substance and some of its compounds are used in toothpastes to slow tooth decay. In many countries it is added to the water supply prior to reaching the consumer. High doses can cause dental fluorosis, nausea, vomiting and even death.

Flashpoint Refers to the lowest temperature at which the vapour above a flammable liquid will ignite on application of a flame. Alcohol has a low flashpoint.

Flavoprotein One of a group of proteins containing riboflavin. They act as oxygen carriers in biological systems.

Foam A coarse dispersion of a gas in a liquid, observed as bubbles. Many modern shaving gels contain low boiling point gases, which boil off and cause foaming when applied to the face. Foam does not actually enhance either cleansing ability or mildness.

Follicle A small cavity in the skin containing the hair root.

Formaldehyde An antimicrobial used in many product groups. It is irritating to the mucous membranes and can be toxic. Its use is banned or restricted in many countries.

Free radicals Molecules or ions with impaired electrons that are extremely reactive. They cause many of the rancidity reactions that occur in natural oils and antioxidants are added to products to prevent this.

Freeze drying The removal of water from a frozen solid.

Fuller's earth An absorptive clay consisting of fine siliceous material, used in face masks to draw out impurities from the skin. It may be used instead of talc.

Fungicide A material that is able to kill at least some types of fungi.

Fungistatic A material inhibiting the growth and multiplication of some types of fungi.

Gas chromatography (also gas liquid chromatography, GLC) A method of analysis often used to help determine the components of essential oils and other liquids.

Gel A suspension of solid and liquid particles that exists as a solid or semi-solid mass.

Gelatin Gelatin is manufactured from the bones and hides of animals by purifying the protein collagen. It is used as a thickener, to form gels and in the manufacture of capsule shells.

Geraniol A fresh-smelling alcohol that exists naturally in many essential oils such as geranium and palmarosa.

Glucose glutamate A reaction product formed from glucose and glutanic acid which is used as a conditioning/moisturising agent. It is essentially non-toxic.

Glycereth The product resulting from the condensation of glycerol with ethylene oxide. It is a humectant to provide moisturising. See also Glycerin.

Glyceryl stearate A white, waxy solid that is prepared by combining glycerol and stearic acid chemically. It is used as an emulsifier and a moisturizing ingredient. It is onsidered non-toxic.

Glycerin A colourless, odourless viscous liquid with a very sweet taste. Known technically as glycerol, it is a form of alcohol that is used as a solvent, sweetener and humectant in cosmetics. It helps to prevent creams from drying out. Glycerin can be manufactured from animal or plant material. It is generally non-toxic and non-irritant.

Glycol stearate Also known as glycol distearate, this is a reaction product of glycol and stearic acid commonly used as an emulsifier in creams. It has no known toxicity.

Glycolic acid An acid used for pH control. It can be extremely irritating to the skin.

Glycols The materials containing the alcohol groups (i.e. OH). They tend to be very thick, humectant liquids which are often used as solubilizers and to impart a moisturizing effect.

Glycyrrhizic acid An acid derived from liquorice root. It has antibacterial properties, which make it particularly suitable for use in deodorants.

Guar hydroxypropyltrimonium chloride A cationic surfactant derived from chemically modified guar gum.

Hardness of water Refers to water containing alkaline earth salts, which prevent formation of a lather with soaps. Detergents can help remove the hardness of water.

Hectorite A mineral found in bentonite clay used as a thickening agent and for its absorption and conditioning properties.

Histamine A chemical released via the body's immune system in response to allergens.

Humectant A substance that reduces water loss from the skin and aids moisturization.

Hydrocarbon A molecule consisting of just hydrogen and carbon. They are generally petrochemical derived and are used as propellants in aerosols and as emollients in cosmetics.

Hydrochloric acid A strong acid used for pH adjustment. It is highly irritant in concentration.

Hydrogenated oil An oil that has hydrogen added to solidify it.

Hydrogen peroxide A chemical used in cosmetics for bleaching and perming hair. It also has antiseptic properties. It is very potent and in concentration can cause damage to the hair shaft and burning on the skin.

Hydrolysed animal protein An animal protein that has been broken down chemically to remove hydrogen and used in toiletries to improve the feel of skin and hair. Some reactions can occur with milk protein.

Hydroscopic Capable of absorbing moisture from the atmosphere.

Hypoallergenic In the strictest sense means without fragrance, but more broadly refers to products that are unlikely to cause skin irritation.

Hydrolysis A decomposition reaction that involves the splitting of water into its ions at the formation of a weak acid or base, or both.

Hydromethylcellulose A chemically modified form of cellulose that is used as a thickening agent.

IFRA The International Fragrance Association, which provides information, recommendations and guidelines on the legislative, toxicological and dermatological aspects of perfumery.

Imidazolidinyl urea An antimicrobial agent, commonly used as a preservative. It can release formaldehyde into formulations if not used correctly. It can cause sensitization but is generally considered to be of low toxicity.

IMS Industrial methylated spirits, generally of ethanol, which has a chemical added to make it unsuitable for internal consumption.

Infusion The liquid resulting from boiling plant material with water in order to extract water-soluble plant components.

Insecticide A material used to control insects. Citronella essential oil provides an excellent natural insecticide.

Insoluble Material that does not dissolve in a solvent.

Iron oxide A pigment used to colour cosmetics.

Irritant Any compound that causes a negative skin reaction on application or sometimes after application.

Isoluitane A propellant used in aerosol products.

Isoprene The smallest building block of terpenes.

Isopropyl myristate A chemically modified fatty acid that has emollient properties. It is generally considered to be non-toxic, although there is concern that its use increases the ability of the skin to absorb other more toxic compounds – nitrosamines, for example.

Kaolin A white powdery clay, also known as china clay, which arises following decomposition of feldspars in granites. It is used in face powder and clay masks for its absorption properties.

Kathon CG The trade name for the preservative octhilinone, which is used as a fungicide and preservative in shampoos and cosmetics. Sensitization is possible.

Keratin A fibrous protein found in hair and nails.

Keralolytic An agent that causes skin shedding and removes surface layers of skin.

Laneth-16 A mixture of ethoxylates produced from lanolin alcohol used for emulsifying and solubilizing. It can be a mild irritant.

Lanolin A preparation of cholesterol and its esters obtained from wool fat. The lanolin is washed off the wool of living sheep. In the past many people thought they were allergic to lanolin; they were actually allergic to the detergent that was used to extract the lanolin from the wool. In recent years only mild detergent is used. Anhydrous lanolin refers to lanolin that does not contain water. Lanolin is an excellent emollient and thickener. It is protective to the skin and well tolerated by people with sensitive skin.

Lanolin alcohol A mixture of alcohols obtained by hydrolysis of lanolin, used for its moisturizing properties.

Lauramide MIPA A non-ionic surfactant used for emulsifying properties. See also Lauric acid.

Laureth 1 to 23 Products of the combination of ethylene oxide with lauryl alcohol to enhance emulsifying properties.

Lauric acid A fatty acid occurring in milk, laurel oil, coconut oil, palm oil and other vegetable oils. It is used to make soaps, detergents and lauryl alcohol.

Lauryl alcohol A fatty alcohol often obtained from coconut oil, used to make anionic surfactants such as sodium laureth sulphate. It has good foaming qualities. It is mildly irritant in concentration but it is non-sensitizing.

Lauryl betaine A synthetic detergent based on vegetable-derived raw materials which is used to create milder formulations when combined with detergents such as sodium lauryl sulphate. See also Lauric alcohol.

Lauryl sulphate Derived from lauryl alcohol, this is used to make detergents as in ammonium lauryl sulphate, sodium lauryl sulphate.

Lecithin An excellent natural emulsifier present in all living organisms but usually commercially derived from the processing of soya oil. It contains a mixture of stearic, palmitic and oleic acid compounds and has antioxidant and emollient properties.

Lethal dose (LD/50) The lethal dose of a substance that, when administered to a group of experimental animals over a period given, causes the death of 50 per cent of them.

Lignin A polymer occurring with cellulose in lignified plant tissues.

Lime soap An insoluble calcium and magnesium fatty acid soap formed when soluble soaps are added to hard water.

Limonene A component of many essential oils. Also manufactured synthetically. Irritant in concentration.

Linalool An alcohol that is a component in many essential oils, such as lavender and coriander.

Linoleic acid An unsaturated fatty acid that occurs in some vegetable oils, especially linseed oil.

129

Lipids Natural substances of a fat-like nature.

Liposomes Artificial microscopic sacs or vesicles used for the introduction of various agents into cells in vitro. They can be manufactured from a variety of substances, including phospholipids. Some manufacturers claim they can be used to deliver certain substances to the underlying layers of the skin.

Litmus A natural colouring matter obtained from lichens used as an indicator of the presence of certain chemicals.

Lake An insoluble pigment obtained by the combination of an organic colouring matter with an inorganic compound. Lakes are used primarily in colour cosmetics.

Lye Potassium or sodium hydroxide, a strong alkaline base found in hair straighteners.

Magnesium aluminium silicate A component of natural clays that is used as a thickener and suspending agent.

Magnesium sulphate See Epsom salts.

Malic acid An acid found in certain herbs and fruits. It has antioxidant and astringent properties.

Medicated products Products that contain active ingredients to produce a specific physiological action.

Melanin The brown pigment of hair, skin and eyes. It arises by oxidation of lyrosine by the action of tyrosinase, especially during exposure to the sun.

Methyl parabens See Parabens.

Mica Silicate compounds used in eye colour cosmetics to create a glittery effect.

Milk A cleanser, emollient, moisturizer and softener, readily absorbed by the skin. Milk is high in protein, calcium and vitamins. Sensitization is possible.

Mineral oil An oil obtained as a by-product of petroleum refinement, frequently used in cosmetics and toiletries such as lipsticks and baby oil for its emollient and lubricant properties. Mineral oil is not readily absorbed by the skin and tends to block the pores. It can be useful in producing barrier creams. It is not considered toxic.

Mucous membranes Thin layers of tissue that line the respiratory, intestinal and genito-urinary tracts. They produce mucus as a protective film. They tend to be more sensitive and permeable to all types of preparations than other areas of skin.

Mud Draws impurities through the skin and removes excess surface oil, dirt and grime. It can also be used to cleanse the hair. Mud packs have long been used for cleansing and therapeutic purposes.

Musk The dried secretion from the sexual glands of the male musk deer. In the past it was much valued for its use in perfumes as a fragrance and fixative. Its use has declined in recent years as it has been replaced with the synthetic musk ambrette.

Myristalkonium chloride A quaternary ammonium compound used as a cationic surfactant in conditioning rinses. It can be irritant to eyes and skin in concentration.

Myristic acid A solid organic acid occurring naturally in many animal and vegetable fats, notably coconut oil. It is combined with potassium to produce a soap with a copious lather. It has no known toxicity.

Myristyl alcohol An emollient prepared from fatty acids and used in creams and lotions. It is non-toxic.

Nail polish A varnish used to colour the nails that is a cocktail of many chemicals, including nitro-cellulose, butyl acetate, toluene, alkyl esters, glycol derivatives, gums, hydrocarbons, lakes and ketones. Nail polish is one of the most toxic and irritant of all cosmetics.

Nail polish remover The main active ingredient in most nail polish removers is acetone, but many commercial formulae also contain conditioning agents. Acetone is a synthetic ingredient that is highly dangerous if taken internally – be sure to wash nails thoroughly after using remover to avoid any being ingested. In fact, acetone is already banned or restricted in many countries.

Natural No official definition exists, but this term generally refers to products that exist in nature and are not further processed.

Natural colouring Food and cosmetic dyes which are unprocessed. The range of colours is limited and they are more prone to fading than synthetic dyes. The accepted natural colourings are less likely to be toxic than synthetic dyes. See also Carmine, Carotene.

Nerol An alcohol found in many essential oils including neroli, lemon grass, orange and rose.

Niacin Vitamin B3.

Nitrosamines Compounds formed by the combination of a secondary amine with an oxide of nitrogen. They are highly carcinogenic in even minute quantities (parts per million). They are found in food products such as cured bacon, beer and also in cosmetics. In formulating products, care must be taken to prevent the formation of nitrosamines by monitoring pH and using antioxidant compounds. Some raw materials by their nature have the potential to cause nitrosamine formation and these must be especially closely monitored when used in formulae.

Non-ionic surfactant A surface active agent that has no electrical charge on it. Examples include polysorbate 20, cetyl stearyl alcohol. They can render formulations much milder.

Nonoxynol-10 A non-ionic emulsifier that is a derivative of phenol. It is irritant in concentration.

Occlusive agent A substance that prevent compounds from leaving a surface. On the skin, oils can act as occlusive agents by preventing the evaporation of water.

Octyl dimethyl PABA See PABA.

Oil Describes a naturally occurring hydrocarbon that can be plant, animal or mineral derived.

Ointment base Available from Neal's Yard Remedies stores; contains de-ionized water, glycerine, polysorbate-20, cetyl stearyl alcohol, beeswax, jojoba oil, methyl parabens and propyl parabens.

Oleakonium chloride A quaternary ammonium compound that is a cationic surfactant with conditioning and antistatic properties.

Oleic acid An emollient with good skin-penetrating properties. Obtained from animal or vegetable fats, it oxidizes rapidly on exposure to the air. It is mildly irritant.

Oleoresin A plant extract consisting of essential oil and resin extracted using a solvent. Oleoresins may then be further diluted using a base oil – for example, benzoin extract, carrot extract.

Oleth 2-20 Oily products derived from fatty alcohols and used as surfactants. They have no known toxicity.

Oleyl alcohol An oily product that is obtained from tallow, fish oil and vegetable oils, for example palm oil. It is used in the manufacture of detergents as an antifoam agent and for its emollient properties. It has no known toxicity.

Opacifying agent A substance used to make cosmetics and toiletries appear opaque and improve their aesthetic appeal.

Organic Describes products that have been certified as grown without the use of artificial pesticides and fertilizers by the Soil Association or other certifying authority.

Oxidation A chemical reaction involving oxygen and causing rancidity to many natural oils. Antioxidants are often added to prevent this happening.

Ozokerite A naturally occurring mineral wax that is used as a thickener. It has no known toxicity.

PABA A water-soluble acid (para-aminobenzoic acid) found in B vitamins and used as a sunscreen agent. Natural PABA is a sensitizer; synthetically produced octyl dimethyl PABA is not.

Pantothenic acid (B5) A B-complex water-soluble vitamin, used in hair and skin-care products for its moisturizing actions. It has no known toxicity.

Parabens Parahydroxybenzoic acid esters used as preservatives in foods, cosmetics and toiletries. They have a broad spectrum antimicrobial action. They are found in nature, but for commercial purposes are synthetically produced. They have a long history of relatively safe use, but like all synthetic preservatives they do have some potential for irritation. Commonly used parabens include methyl parabens, propyl parabens, ethyl parabens and butyl parabens. Effective levels are 0.1–0.3 per cent concentration in the overall product. See also Propyl parabens.

Paraffin wax Wax derived from petrochemicals, used as a moisturizer and thickener.

Patch test Describes the technique of applying a small amount of a product prior to full use to see if any allergic reaction occurs. The best places to try a patch test are on the inside of the elbow or, if that is not appropriate, the inside of the wrist. Leave at least two hours for each test. Doing a patch test is strongly advisable prior to buying/trying a new product for anyone with sensitive skin.

Pearlizing agent See Opacifying agent.

Pectin The dried extract of various fruit rinds or vegetables, used as a natural thickener.

PEG derivatives Derivatives of polyethylene glycol, which is prepared from ethylene oxide and water, dihydroxyethane or diethylene glycol plus a base. The amount of ethylene oxide present will dictate the water solubility. These are used as humectants, solubilisers and moisturising agents. PEG products can be combined with oils such as castor oil (eg. PEG 20 Castor Oil) and lanolin to produce a range of non-ionic surfactants which can be used as emulsifiers and conditioners. PEG is usually written with a number after it, for example PEG 24, the number referring to the viscosity; the lower the number the more liquid the product. They are not considered toxic. Those with a higher number (lower molecular level), for example PEG 200-400, may be sensitisers.

Perfume A product used for fragrancing the body, generally based on a combination of fragrant oils with alcohol. Throughout history essential oils and flower waters have been used as perfume materials, though since the 1920s most famous perfumes also include synthetic fragrances. Perfume or fragrance is often the most likely ingredient in a product to cause sensitization; hence hypoallergenic products are without fragrance. Eau de parfum is highly concentrated, eau de toilette less so.

Petroleum jelly (Petrolatum, Vaseline) A salve-like material derived from petroleum, which is used as a lubricant and emollient in many cosmetics and toiletries. It is not considered toxic. Sensitization is possible.

Phenoxyethanol An antimicrobial agent (preservative) often used in combination with parabens. It is manufactured by combining phenol (coal tar derived) with ethylene oxide. It is irritant at high concentrations and sensitization is possible.

Phosphoric acid Used for pH adjustments of products. Irritant in concentration, it is not considered toxic in cosmetic use.

Phytosterols Fatty alcohols that are derived from plants.

Phytotherapy The using of plants and herbs for their therapeutic value.

Polyacrylamide A polymer produced by combination of acrylamide and sodium acrylate that is used as a thickener and additive in tanning products and nail polish. It is toxic and irritant.

Polymer Whenever many small molecules are combined the result is called a polymer. Examples include plastics and animal tissue. In cosmetics it generally refers to a group of non-ionic surfactants based on fatty acid esters of Sorbiton that are used as foaming, cleansing and dispersing agents.

Polyquaternium companiol A synthetic polymer that is combined with ammonium to produce a positively charged nitrogen, rendering it a cationic surfactant. They are used in hair-care products because of their substantivity to hair. See also Quaternary ammonium compound.

Polysorbates 1-85 Products of the combination of lauric acid with sorbitol, which is condensed with ethylene oxide to render it water-soluble. They are generally considered mild and non-toxic. Their main functions are as solubilizers and emulsifiers.

Preservative A substance added to products to prevent their deterioration. Bacteria and fungi will grow in any product with a significant water content. Preservatives are added to inhibit (bacteriostatic) or kill (antibiotic) those microbes that would otherwise cause spoilage. To have a realistic shelf life, commercially manufactured products contain preservatives; otherwise products must be kept in the refrigerator and replaced every few days.

Propane A propellant used in aerosols.

Propolis A substance produced by bees to protect their hive from viral or bacterial attack. Propolis has a preservative and antibiotic action. It is available as a tincture and may be combined into cosmetic formulations.

Propylene glycol A colourless, almost odourless liquid, synthetically produced. It is used in perfumes and flavourings and as a solvent, humectant and moisturizing ingredient in a wide range of cosmetics and toiletries. Sensitization is possible.

Propyl parabens A commonly used broad-spectrum

preservative. Recent evidence suggests that people with certain types of cancer produce an excess of propyl parabens and due to this link the popularity of this substance is declining. There is no evidence to date that propyl parabens causes cancer. See also Parabens.

Protein Building blocks of the human body, which are composed of a combination of amino acids. Keratin, which makes up the hair, is an example.

Quaternary ammonium compound A compound based on ammonium salts where the hydrogen atoms have been replaced by other chemical groups. These compounds are cationic and can be combined with other materials to provide a range of chemical functions, mainly preservatives and surfactants. Examples are Quaternarium 1-30 and Benzalkonium chloride. Many are irritant in concentration. Sensitization is possible.

Resorcinol A synthetically derived alcohol that is used in dandruff shampoos to prevent itching; it also acts as a preservative and reduces skin greasiness. It is a known sensitizer and is irritant in concentration.

Retinoids Derivatives of vitamin A, used in anti-ageing creams and acne treatments. They are toxic in concentration.

Rosin The residue left after distilling off the volatile oil from the oleoresin obtained from *Pinus palustris* and other species of pine trees. It is used in cosmetics and toiletries in soaps, lacquers and depilatory waxes. Sensitization is possible.

Rum Alcohol produced from the distillation of fermented molasses or sugar cane. Rum reduces the production of oil by the sweat glands and is a traditional hair tonic, especially for greasy hair.

Salicylic acid This occurs naturally as methyl salicylate – for example, in oil of wintergreen, from which it can be obtained by treatment with alcoholic potassium hydroxide. The synthetic version, which is more often used commercially, is used in cosmetics as an antiseptic and preservative and for treating acne. Sensitization is possible.

Salt See Sodium chloride.

Saponification The process used in soap-making whereby an oil or fat is reacted with a strong base, for example caustic soda, to produce a soap.

Saponins A group of sugar-based substances forming solutions that foam on shaking. Saponins occur naturally, for example in soapwort herb and quillaja bark, and are also produced synthetically. They are used in cosmetics and drinks for their foaming properties.

SD alcohol An alcohol that has been denatured by the addition of a compound that renders it undrinkable.

Sensitizer A product that causes an allergic reaction. Initial exposure to the product may not cause a noticeable reaction, but subsequent or repeated exposure may cause a severe inflammatory response.

Shellac A resinous substance excreted by various insects on to trees, used as a lacquer and binder. Sensitization is possible.

Silicone A widely used group of oils and compounds derived from the mineral silica. Silicones are water repellent and very stable. There is no known toxicity when used externally.

Silicone derivatives These products, based on silicone, are used in hair-care and skin-care products. Their use in hair care is becoming less popular because they have a tendency to cause build-up. They have no known toxicity.

Simethicone A mixture of dimethicone and silica, used as a conditioning agent. It has no known toxicity.

Sodium ascorbate Salt form of vitamin C used as an antioxidant and preservative in cosmetics.

Sodium benzoate An antiseptic and preservative used in food and cosmetics. It is non-toxic externally.

Sodium bicarbonate An alkaline substance used in deodorants and toothpastes for its absorption properties and as a pH neutralizer.

Sodium borate See Borax.

Sodium carbonate Known as washing soda when hydrated. It is used in glass, soap and chemical detergents. Sensitization is possible.

Sodium chloride Common salt, used as an astringent and antiseptic. It also appears in some cosmetic formulations, for example shampoos, as a thickener. It is considered non-toxic and non-irritant externally in dilution.

Sodium citrate Salt of citric acid, used medicinally as a blood anticoagulant and in cosmetics as a buffering agent and sequestrant. It is non-toxic externally.

Sodium hydroxide See Caustic soda.

Sodium lactate A thick colourless liquid that is a natural component of the skin's upper layers, used for its moisturizing properties.

Sodium monofluorophosphate Used in toothpastes to provide fluoride to prevent tooth decay. See Fluoride.

Sodium lauryl sulphate A synthetic detergent of which the origins may be plant (coconut and palm kernel oil) or animal. It is one of the most common ingredients used in shampoos and toothpastes for its foaming and detergent properties. It can be irritant in concentration, but correct formulation renders them functional with low irritancy.

Sodium laureth sulphate Similar to sodium lauryl sulphate except that it contains ethylene oxide to render it more water-soluble and consequently milder. See also Ethoxylate.

Sodium silicate A mineral-derived component often found in clays such as kaolin and bentonite.

Sodium tetraborate See Borax.

Soft detergents Detergents that are biodegradable.

Solvent A substance used to dissolve solute or extract components from solid material.

Solvent extraction The removal of soluble material from a solid mixture by means of a solvent or the removal of components from a liquid mixture by use of a solvent with which the liquid is unmixable, or nearly so.

Sorbic acid Obtained from the berries of the rowan tree (*Sorbus aucuparia*) or synthetically manufactured, sorbic acid is used as a preservative, binder and humectant in cosmetics. It is non-toxic and non-irritant in dilution. Sensitization is possible.

Sorbitan fatty acid esters Mixtures of fatty acids with esters of sorbitol, for example sorbitan oleate, sorbitan stearate. They have wide-ranging use in cosmetics as emulsifying, stabilizing, surfactant and thickening agents. They are generally considered to be non-toxic and non-irritant, although they may cause blackheads in susceptible individuals.

Sorbitan oleate A reaction product of oleic acid and sorbitol, used as a thickener and emollient. It has been reported to cause blackheads.

Sorbitol Alcohol derivative of glucose used as a humectant, binder and sweetener in cosmetics. It occurs naturally in certain fruits. It is non-toxic externally.

SPF Sun protection factor, an indicator of the degree of sun protection that a sunscreen offers. As a rule, for each SPF number 20 minutes of sun protection is offered by correct use of the product. Low SPF products tend to be in the SPF range of 1–6; medium SPF 7–11; and high 12 to 30+. There is some debate as to whether an SPF over 20 does in fact offer greater protection. The SPF rating applies to UVB protection only. See also Sunscreens.

Squalene A component of various animal and vegetable oils, commercially extracted from shark-liver oil, which has lubricant and fixative properties. It has no known toxicity.

Starch A sugar polymer derived from plant sources, used in cosmetics for its absorbent and soothing properties. Sensitization to various forms of starch is possible.

Stearalkonium chloride See Quaternary ammonium compound.

Steareth compounds Compounds produced by ethoxylation of stearyl alcohol, which are used as solubilizers and coemulsifiers.

Stearic acid A waxy, fatty acid that can be derived from tallow and other animal fats, but also from cocoa butter and other vegetable fats. It is used as an emulsifier and emollient in soaps, creams and lotions. It is non-toxic. Sensitization is unusual but possible.

Stratum corneum The outer hardened layer of the skin.

Sunscreens Substances used to block out the sun's burning rays. Sunscreens may act in two main ways: chemical sunscreens, for example PABA, which refract the sun's rays; and physical sunscreens, for example titanium dioxide, which block the sun's rays from reaching the skin. Sunscreens are also divided into those that protect against UVB light, which causes immediate burning (and this is what the SPF system is based on); and those that protect against UVA light, which is thought to cause longer term but less immediately obvious damage and premature ageing. See also SPF.

Surfactant A substance with the ability to reduce the surface tension at the interface between two unlike surfaces. Soap is an example, as are all detergents. Amphoteric surfactants have both a positive (cationic) group and a negative (anionic) group. The final pH of a product will dictate which group is more dominant. At an intermediate pH, both forms are present. At a pH of less than 7 the cationic group is more prevalent, and at a pH of over 7 the anionic group is more prevalent. They tend to be very mild and are often found in baby products. Anionic surfactants are negatively charged surface active agents used widely in shampoo and foaming baths as the primary cleansing agent. These are chemically produced, although the raw materials used to produce them can be vegetable, animal or mineral derived. Examples include ammonium lauryl sulphate, sodium laureth sulphate. Cationic surfactants are detergents of which the ions are positively charged. They are used mainly in conditioners. See also Detergent.

Talc Magnesium silicate, obtained by mining, also known as talcum powder or French chalk. It has soothing, absorbtive and anti-chafing properties and is used in body powders and as a base for many colour cosmetics. It is irritant if inhaled. There is some evidence of toxicity if it is absorbed through the skin.

Tallow Fat obtained from the fatty tissue of animals (usually cows and sheep), used to make some soaps, emulsifiers and glycerol.

Tannins A large group of substances found in plants. They are used for their astringency.

Terpinol One of the active components of tea tree oil, also found in other oils.

Tincture An extract that has been prepared using alcohol and water to extract plant components.

Titanium dioxide A mineral salt that is used as a white pigment in makeup and as a physical sunblock in high SPF sunscreen lotions. It has no known external toxicity.

Tocopherol A form of vitamin E, usually extracted from soya oil. It is used as an antioxidant in a wide range of cosmetics and toiletries. It is non-toxic and non-sensitizing. Also known as vitamin E acetate.

Tragacanth A gum which is used as a thickener. Sensitization is possible.

Triclosan A white powder which is used as an antimicrobial and deodorant. It is a known sensitizer.

Triethanolamine A frequently used dispersing agent and emulsifier. It is irritant in concentration and sensitization is possible.

Urea A product of protein metabolism present in urine. It is used in cosmetics and toiletries as an anti-septic and preservative. It has no known toxicity externally.

Vegetable oil An oil extracted from a plant as opposed to an animal or mineral oil.

Vinegar Dilute acetic acid, used as an astringent and pH adjuster.

Viscosity Degree of pourability or stickiness. A highly viscous product is thick and sticky, for example treacle, while a product with low viscosity is readily pourable and 'thin' – water, for example.

Wax Fatty acid esters that are water-repellent and have plasticity.

Wetting agent A substance that increases the spreading of a liquid by reducing the tension between two surfaces.

Wool wax See Lanolin.

Xanthan gum Also known as corn sugar gum, this is a polysaccharide produced from bacteria (*Xanthomonas campestris*) fermented with a carbohydrate. It is used in food and cosmetics as a thickener, emulsifier and stabiliser. It has no known toxicity.

Zinc oxide A soft white powder used as a white pigment. It has antimicrobial, preservative and water-repellent properties. It is frequently used in baby creams to prevent nappy rash and is also effective as a sunscreen. It is not considered toxic in cosmetic use.

Zinc pyrithione A synthetic anti-dandruff active ingredient. It is a sensitizer and possible irritant.

Tinctures

To make tinctures (see page 21), follow the ratios between the plant material and the water/100% alcohol mixture shown in the wt/vol column. The proportion of alcohol to water required is given in the %alc column.

Latin Name	Common Name	wt/vol	% alc
Achillea millefolium	Yarrow Herb	1:5	25
Acorus calamus	Sweet Flag Root	1:5	60
Aesculus hippocastaneum	Horsechestnut	1:5	25
Alchemilla arvensis	Parsley Piert Herb	1:5	25
Alchemilla vulgaris	Lady's Mantle Herb	1:5	25
Aletris farinosa	Unicorn Root	1:5	25
Aloe ferox	Cape Aloes	1:40	45
Alpinia officinarum	Galangal Rhizome	1:5	25
Althaea officinalis	Marsh Mallow	1:5	25
Ammi visnaga	Khella Fruits	1:5	25
Anemone pulsatilla	Pasque Flower Herb	1:10	25
Angelica archangelica	Angelica	1:5	45
Apium graveolens	Celery Seed	1:4	60
Arctium lappa	Burdock Root	1:5	25
Arctostaphylos uva-ursi	Bearberry Leaf	1:5	25
Armoracia rusticana	Horseradish Root	1:10	45
Arnica montana	Arnica Flower	1:10	45
Artemisia abrotanum	Southernwood Herb	1:10	45
Artemisia absinthium	Wormwood Herb	1:10	45
Artemisia vulgaris	Mugwort Herb	1:10	45
Asclepias tuberosa	Pleurisy Root	1:10	25
Avena sativa	Oats	1:5	25
Baptisia tinctoria	Wild Indigo Root	1:10	60
Berberis vulgaris	Barberry Bark	1:5	25
Betula pendula	Birch Leaf	1:5	25
Borago officinalis	Borage Herb	1:5	25
Calendula officinalis	Marigold Flower	1:5	25
Capsella bursa-pastoris	Shepherd's Purse Herb	1:5	25
Capsicum frutescens	Cayenne Fruits	1:20	60
Carum carvi	Caraway Seed	1:5	45
Cedrella asiatica	Toona	1:5	25
Cephaelis ipecacuanha BP 1983	Ipecacuanha Root	1:10	90
Chamaelirion luteum	False Unicorn Root	1:10	90
Chamaclemum nobile	Roman Chamomile	1:5	45
Chamomilia recutita	German Chamomile	1:5	45
Chondrus crispus	Irish Moss alga	1:5	25
Cinnamomum zeylanicum	Cinnamon Bark	1:5	45
Cola nitida	Cola Nut	1:5	25

Latin Name	Common Name	wt/vol	% alc
Collinsonia canadensis	Stone Root	1:5	25
Commiphora myrrha	Myrrh Oleo Gum Resin	1:5	90
Echinacea angustifolia	Coneflower Root	1:5	45
Eleutherococcus	Siberian Ginseng Root	1:5	25
Equisetum arvense	Horsetail Herb	1:5	25
Erythraea centaurium	Centaury Herb	1:5	25
Eschscholtzia californica	Californian Poppy	1:5	45
Eucalyptus globulus	Eucalyptus Leaf	1:5	45
Euphorbia hirta	Euphorbia Herb	1:5	60
Euphrasia species	Eyebright Herb	1:5	25
Foeniculum vulgare	Fennel Seed	1:5	45
Fucus vesiculosus	Bladderwrack	1:2	25
Fumaria officinalis	Fumitory Herb	1:5	25
Galega officinalis	Goat's Rue Herb	1:5	25
Galium aparine	Cleavers Herb	1:5	25
Gentiana lutea	Gentian Root	1:5	45
Geranium maculatum Radix	Cranesbill Root	1:5	25
Geum urbanum	Avens Herb	1:5	25
Ginkgo biloba	Maidenhair Tree Leaf	1:5	25
Glechoma hederacea	Ground Ivy Herb	1:5	25
Grindelia camporum	Grindelia Herb	1:10	25
Guaiacum officinale	Lignum vitae Resin	1:5	90
Hamamelis virginiana	Witch Hazel	1:5	25
Harpagophytum procumbens	Devil's Claw Tuber	1:5	25
Humulus lupulus	Hops Strobiles	1:5	60
Hydrangea arborescens	Hydrangea Root	1:5	25
Hydrastis canadensis	Golden Seal Root	1:10	60
Hypericum perforatum	St John's Wort Herb	1:5	45
Hyssopus officinalis	Hyssop Herb	1:5	45
Jateorhiza palmala	Calumba Root	1:10	60
Juglans cinerea	Butternut Bark	1:5	25
Juniperus communis	Juniper Berry	1:5	45
Lactuca virosa	Wild Lettuce Leaf	1:5	25
Lamium album	White Deadnettle	1:5	25

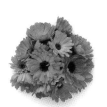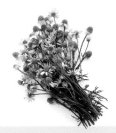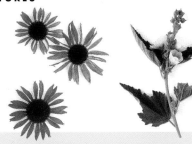

Latin Name	Common Name	wt/vol	% alc
Larrea mexicana	Chapparal	1:5	25
Lavandula augustifolia	Lavender Flower	1:5	45
Leptandra virginica	Black Root	1:5	70
Lycopus virginicus	Bugleweed Herb	1:5	25
Mahonia aquifolium	Oregon Grape Root	1:5	25
Marsdenia condurango	Condurango Bark	1:5	45
Matricaria recutita	German Chamomile	1:5	45
Medicago sativa	Alfalfa/Lucerne Herb	1:5	25
Melilotus officinalis	Melilot	1:5	25
Melissa officinalis	Lemon Balm Herb	1:5	45
Mentha x piperita	Peppermint herb	1:5	45
Ononis spinosa	Restharrow Root	1:5	45
Paneax ginseng	Korean Ginseng Root	1:5	25
Parietaria diffusa	Pellitory of the wall Herb	1:5	25
Passiflora incarnata	Passion Flower Herb	1:8	25
Peumus boldus	Boldo Leaf	1:10	60
Phytolacca americana	Poke Root	1:5	45
Pilosella officinalis	Mouse Ear Hawkweed	1:5	25
Pimpinella anisum	Aniseed	1:5	45
Piper methysticum	Kava Kava Root	1:5	25
Piscidia erythrina	Jamaican Dogwood	1:5	30
Plantago lanceolata	Ribwort Leaf	1:5	25
Polygonum bistorta	Bistort Root	1:5	25
Populus tremuloides	White Poplar Bark	1:5	25
Potentilla tormentilla	Tormentil Rhizome	1:5	25
Prunus serotina	Wild Cherry Bark	1:5	25
Pulmonaria officinalis	Lungwort Leaf	1:5	25
Quercus robur	Oak Bark	1:5	25
Ranunculus ficaria	Pilewort Herb	1:5	25
Rhamnus purshianus	Cascara Bark	1:5	25
Rheum officinale	Rhubarb Root	1:5	25
Rhus aromatica	Sweet Surmac Root	1:5	25
Rosmarinus officinalis	Rosemary Leaf	1:5	45
Rubus idaeus	Raspberry Leaf	1:5	25
Rumex crispus	Yellow Dock Root	1:5	25
Ruta graveolens	Rue Herb	1:5	25

Latin Name	Common Name	wt/vol	% alc
Salvia officinalis	Red Sage	1:5	45
Sambucus nigra	Elderflower	1:5	25
Sanguinaria canadensis	Bloodroot Rhizome	1:5	60
Sarothamnus scoparius	Broom Tops	1:5	25
Senna angustifolia	Senna Pod & Leaf	1:5	45
Serenoa serrulata	Saw Palmetto Berry	1:5	90
Smilax species	Sarsparilla Root	1:5	25
Solidago virgaurea	Golden Rod Herb	1:5	25
Stachys betonica	Wood Betony Herb	1:5	25
Stellaria media	Chickweed Herb	1:5	25
Stillingia sylvatica	Queen's Delight Root	1:5	45
Symphytum officinale	Comfrey	1:10	25
Tabebuia impetiginosa	Lapacho	1:5	45
Tanacetum vulgare	Tansy Herb	1:5	45
Tanacetum parthenium .	Feverfew Herb	2:5	25
Taraxacum officinale	Dandelion	1:5	25
Teucrium chamaedrys	Germander Herb	1:5	25
Teucrium scorodonia	Wood Sage Herb	1:5	25
Thuja occidentalis	Thuja Tips	1:10	60
Thymus vulgaris	Thyme Herb	1:5	45
Tilia europaea	Lime Flower	1:5	25
Trifolium pratense	Red Clover Flower	1:10	25
Trillium erectum	Birthroot	1:5	45
Turnera diffusa	Damiana Leaf	1:5	60
Tussilago farfara	Coltsfoot Leaf	1:5	25
Ulmus fulva	Slippery Elm Bark	1:5	25
Urginea maritima	Squill Bulb	1:10	60
Urtica dioica	Stinging Nettle Herb	1:5	25
Verbascum thapsus	Mullein Leaf	1:5	25
Viburnum opulus	Crampbark	1:5	25
Viburnum prunifolium	Black Haw Bark	1:5	25
Vinca major	Greater Periwinkle Herb	1:5	25
Viola odorata	Sweet Violet Leaf	1:5	25
Viola tricolor	Heartsease Herb	1:5	25
Vitex agnus castus	Chasteberry	1:5	25
Zea mays	Corn Silk Stigmata	1:5	25
Zingiber officinale	Ginger Root	1:2	90

Useful Addresses

SUPPLIERS

When purchasing ingredients, it is essential to choose products of good quality. Herbs should be fresh and, where possible, organically grown. Essential oils must be pure and of natural origin. Synthetic oils will not produce satisfactory results and may be damaging.

Most of the products mentioned in this book (essential oils, herbs, homoeopathic supplies and 'make your own' ingredients), as well as a large selection of books and literature, are available from branches of Neal's Yard Remedies. A mail order service is also available: telephone 0161 831 7875.

NEAL'S YARD REMEDIES STORES

Neal's Yard Remedies
15 Neal's Yard
Covent Garden
London WC2H 9DP
Tel 0171 379 7222

Neal's Yard Remedies
Chelsea Farmers Market
Sydney Street
London SW3 6NR
Tel 0171 351 6380

Neal's Yard Remedies
9 Elgin Crescent
London W11 2JA
Tel 0171 727 3998

Neal's Yard Remedies
68 Chalk Farm Road
Camden
London NW1 8AN
Tel 0171 284 2039

Neal's Yard Remedies
The Glades Shopping
Centre, Bromley
Kent BR1 1DD
Tel 0181 313 9898

Neal's Yard Remedies
2a Kensington Gardens
Brighton BN1 4AL
Tel 01273 601464

Neal's Yard Remedies
5 Golden Cross
Cornmarket Street
Oxford OX1 3EU
Tel 01865 245436

Neal's Yard Remedies
31 King Street
Manchester M2 6AA
Tel 0161 831 7875

Neal's Yard Remedies
126 Whiteladies Road
Clifton
Bristol BS8 2RP
Tel 0117 946 6034

Neal's Yard Remedies
26 Lower Goat Lane
Norwich NR2 1EL
Tel 01603 766681

JAPAN

Neal's Yard Remedies
PO Box 150
AHMS 1F
1-18-4 Ebisu Nishi
Shibuya-Ku
Tokyo 150
Japan

BRAZIL

Neal's Yard Remedies
Rua Melo Alves 383
Cerqueira Cezar
Sao Paulo – SP
CEP 01417 010
Brazil

OTHER HERB SUPPLIERS

G Baldwin & Co
171-73 Walworth Road
London SE17 1RW
Tel 0171 703 5550

Culpeper Ltd
Head Office
Handstock Road
Linton
Cambridge CB1 6NJ
Tel 01223 891196
(ring for branches)

Napier & Sons
18 Nicholson Street
Edinburgh EH8 9DJ

OTHER ESSENTIAL OIL SUPPLIERS

Tisserand Aromatherapy
Newtown Road
Hove
Sussex
BN3 7BA
Tel 01273 325666

OTHER HOMOEOPATHIC SUPPLIERS

Ainsworths
38 New Cavendish Street
London W1M 7LH
Tel 0171 935 5330

Helios
97 Camden Road
Tunbridge Wells
Kent TN1 2QR
Tel 01892 537254

Weleda
Heanor Road
Ilkeston
Derbyshire DE7 8DR
Tel 01602 303151

EQUIPMENT SUPPLIES

Most of the equipment can be bought from good chemists, wine-making specialists, kitchen equipment and department stores. One of the most comprehensively stocked chemists is:

John Bell & Croyden
52-54 Wigmore Street
London W1H 0AU
Tel 0171 935 5555

For further information regarding herbs, herb growing, events and so on, contact:

The Herb Society
134 Buckingham Palace Road
London SW1W 9SA
0171 823 5583

FINDING A NATURAL HEALTH PRACTITIONER

Aromatherapy
Organisations Council
3 Latymer Close
Braybrooke
Market Harborough
Leicester LE16 8LN
Tel 01858 434242

Bach Flower Remedies
Dr Edward Bach Centre
Mount Vernon
Sotwell
Wallingford
Oxfordshire OX10 0PZ
Tel 01491 834678

British Acupuncture
Council
Park House
206-208 Latimer Road
London W10 6RE
Tel 0181 964 0222

British Chiropractic
Association
Equity House
29 Whitley Street
Reading RG2 0E9
Tel 01734 757557

British Herbal Medicine
Association
Sun House
Church Street
Stroud
Gloucestershire
GL5 1JL

British Massage Therapy
Council
Greenbank House
65a Adelphi Street
Preston PR1 7BH
Tel 01772 881063

British Register of
Complementary Medicine
Institute of Complementary
Medicine
PO Box 194
London SE16 1QZ
Tel 0171 237 5165

Council for Nutrition
Education & Therapy
34 Wadham Road
London SW15 2LR

Craniosacral Therapy
Association
8 Warren Road
Colliers Wood
London SW19 2HX
Tel 0181 543 4969

General Council & Register
of Naturopaths
Goswell House
2 Goswell Road
Street
Somerset BS16 0JG
Tel 01458 840072

Healing Herbs of Dr Bach
PO Box 65
Hereford HR2 0UW
Tel 01873 890218

International Association of
Clinical Iridologists
853 Finchley Road
London NW11 8LX

Kinesiology Federation
PO Box 7891
Wimbledon
London SW19 1ZB
Tel 0181 545 9255

National Federation of
Spiritual Healers
Old Manor Farm Studio
Church Street
Sunbury-on-Thames
Middlesex TW16 6RG
Tel 0891 616080

National Institue of Medical
Herbalists
56 Longbrook Street
Exeter
Devon EX4 6AH

National Register of
Hypnotherapists and
Psychotherapists
12 Cross Street
Nelson
Lancashire BB9 7EN
Tel 01282 699378

Natural Medicines Society
Edith Lewis House
Ilkeston
Derbyshire DE7 8EJ
Tel 01602 329454

Osteopathic Information
Service
PO Box 2074
Reading
Berkshire RG1 4YR
Tel 01734 512051

Reflexology Organizations
Council
92 Sheering Road
Old Harlow
Essex CM17 0JW
Tel 01279 429060

Register of Chinese Herbal
Medicine
PO Box 400
Wembley
Middlesex HA5 9NZ

The Shiatsu Society
5 Foxcote
Wokingham
Berkshire RG11 3PG
Tel 01734 730836

Society of Homoeopaths
2 Artizan Road
Northampton
NN1 4HU
Tel 01604 21400

Society of Teachers of
Alexander Technique
266 Fulham Road
London SW10 9EL
Tel 0171 351 0828

United Kingdom
Homoeopathic Medical
Association
6 Livingstone Road
Gravesend
Kent DA12 5DZ
Tel 01474 560336

MISCELLANEOUS

British Association of
Homoeopathic Veterinary
Surgeons
Chinham House
Stanford in the Vale
Faringdon
Oxfordshire SN7 8NQ

British Complementary
Medicine Association
39 Prestbury Road
Pittville
Cheltenham GL52 2PT
Tel 01242 226770

British Homoeopathic
Dental Association
12 Wellington Road
Watford
Hertfordshire
WD1 1QW

Council for
Complementary &
Alternative Medicine
179 Gloucester Place
London NW1 6DX
Tel 0171 724 9103

Institute for
Complementary Medicine
PO Box 194
London SE16 1QZ

AUSTRALIA

Association of Massage
Therapists
18a Spit Road
Mosman
NSW 2088
Tel 969 8445

Association of Remedial
Masseurs
22 Stuart Street
Ryde
NSW 2112
Tel 878 2159

Australian Federation of
Homoeopaths
21 Bulah Close
Berowra Heights
NSW 2082
Tel (02) 456 3602

Australian Natural
Therapists Association
PO Box 522
Sutherland
NSW 2232
Tel (02) 521 2063

Australian Traditional
Medicine Society
120 Blaxland Road
Ryde
NSW 2112
Tel (02) 808 2825

Herb Society of Western
Australia
149 Bradford Street
Coolbinia
Western Australia 6050
Tel (09) 444 5328

National Herbalists'
Association of Australia
PO Box 65
Kingsgrove
NSW 2208
Tel (02) 787 4523

USA

American Chiropractic
Association
1701 Clarendon Blvd
Arlington
VA 24203
Tel 703 276 8800

American Osteopathic
Association
142 E Ontario Street
Chicago
IL 60611
Tel 312 280 5800

Flower Essence Society
PO Box 1769
Nevada City
CA 95969
Tel 916 265 9163

Flower Remedies of Dr
Bach
Dr Edward Bach Healing
Society
644 Merrick Road
Lynbrook
NY 11563
Tel 516 593 2206

National Center for
Homoeopathy
801 N Fairfax Street
Alexandria
VA 22314
Tel 703 548 7790

TRAINING IN NATURAL MEDICINE

UK

College of Homoeopathy
Regent's College
Inner Circle
Regents Park
London NW1 4NW
Tel 0171 487 7416

College of Practical
Homoeopathy
422 Hackney Road
London E2 7SY
0171 613 5468

General Council & Register
of Consultant Herbalists
18 Sussex Square
Brighton
East Sussex
BN2 5AA

London School of
Aromatherapy
PO Box 780
London
NW5 1DY
Tel 0171 267 6717

International Institute of
Reflexology
15 Hartfield Close
Tonbridge
Kent TN10 4JP
Tel 01732 350629

The School of
Phytotherapy
Bucksteep Manor
Bodle Street Green
Hailsham
East Sussex BN27 4RJ
Tel 01323 833812

Tisserand Institute
65 Church Road
Hove
East Sussex BN3 2BD
Tel 01273 206640

UK College for
Complementary Healthcare
Studies
Exmoor Street
London W10 6DZ
Tel 0181 964 1205

AUSTRALIA

Australasian College of
Natural Therapies
620 Harris Street
Ultimo
NSW 2007
Tel (02) 212 6699

Australian Academy of
Osteopathy
7th Floor
235 Macquarie Street
Sydney
NSW 2000
Tel 233 1655

USA

California School of Herbal
Studies
PO Box 39
Forestville
C 95436
Tel 707 887 7457

East West Herb Courses
c/o Michael Tierra
Box 712
Santa Cruz
CA 950061

Index